To

Sarah

Thanks for bringing Glitter
into my life

Nikki

I'M ILL YOU KNOW

by

NIKKI COOMBS

authorHOUSE®

AuthorHouse™ UK Ltd.
500 Avebury Boulevard
Central Milton Keynes, MK9 2BE
www.authorhouse.co.uk
Phone: 08001974150

This book is a work of non-fiction. Unless otherwise noted,
the author and the publisher make no explicit guarantees
as to the accuracy of the information contained in
this book and in some cases, names of people and
places have been altered to protect their privacy.

First published by AuthorHouse 10/23/2007
ISBN: 978-1-4343-3582-1 (sc)

Printed in the United States of America
Bloomington, Indiana

This book is printed on acid-free paper.

THIS BOOK IS DEDICATED TO

Trevor for being there unconditionally, and facing cancer along side me.

Becky and Vicky, you are the best kids a mum and dad could wish for.

All my family and friends, who have been there with me through the good, the bad, and the ugly times. It would be difficult to name all of you, but you know who you are. There are no words of thanks that could repay the support and love you have given me, so I hope you like reading!

The doctors and nurses, I thank you for your honesty, care and for laughing with me.

Anyone who is facing the dreaded 'c' word. We all have choices in this world. Sometimes these choices are forced upon us. This was my choice; to cry and die or live and laugh, you choose!

INTRODUCTION

Most doctors aren't patients. Doctors do interact with patients, they try to understand them, treat them, and sometimes share with them truly privileged conversations. But doctors don't live in their patient's world, they only get glimpses of it, and these are glimpses chosen, extracted and edited by the patient. These extracts help doctors: at root, they can help doctors diagnose patients, they can help them empathise with their patients, and they can help them come to joint decisions with patients. The stories patients tell doctors help doctors understand - a bit - what it is like to be them. But they're only snapshots. How much greater would doctors understanding of patients be, if we were able to live in their world, albeit vicariously, for a little longer?

And how might relatives, friends and carers understand how their "patient" was dealing with a serious illness? In some ways, the carer's roles are not dissimilar to those of doctors and nurses: they will see glimpses, but possibly more prolonged, profound, and problematic ones. Could carers also benefit from living in the world of a seriously ill person for a while, to help them cope with a similar experience in their own lives?

This book presents us all a (literally) unique opportunity to live in Nicola's world for a while. Nicola's is a kingdom ruled, for the period of her life threatening illness, by a rare tumour, with its attendant hospital visits, meetings with doctors and nurses, lumbar punctures and major operations . But it is a world, which, for Nicola, carries on in a disarmingly normal way, almost like a parallel universe: her carpet gets soaked, she goes to the theatre and visits a pantomime. Nicola lives simultaneously at the edge of the human predicament, and right at the centre of her beautiful, normal life.

So, what do we learn? Doctors and nurses don't often talk about their patients being brave – but this is what percolates through every sentence of Nicola's narrative. Doctors and nurses might think their patients are funny, but, again, would rarely discuss it amongst themselves. In her story, Nicola draws upon her irrepressible sense of humour to keep her sane, to make sense of what is senseless, to survive what is recklessly destructive. And we learn that Nicola is generous – to her carers (in spite of her younger doctors trotting in one by one asking exactly the same questions), to her partner Trevor, and delightfully, to herself. Carers might not think that, often, really ill people worry about them – like Nicola does, in one or two truly touching insights into how her partner Trevor is dealing with her predicament – including switching the SatNav voice from Jane to Tim.

Will doctors and nurses, will other patients and carers benefit from reading Nicola's account? Oh, just read on and find out!

Kieran Sweeney
The Foxhayes Practice
Exwick
Exeter.

So it's 4:21AM on the 23rd of September 2006, pouring down with rain and maybe not the best time to start writing this but what the hell! I would like to blame Kieran, my doctor I know it is not his fault but he suggested writing this thing, I am not sure what to call it yet!!

I have woken up at 3:30 am with my jaw and teeth aching and my fists sore and I need to punch someone's lights out. Not sure who that someone is and anyway it really does not matter because I have CANCER.

I want to rip the cancer or choriocarcinoma to be precise out of me and slam it on the professor's desk and say you have it because I sure don't want it. In fact just at this moment there are a lot of things that I don't want;

I don't want to be bought a Sat Nav so we can find Charing Cross hospital. I want to go to places that I have not been to yet but I'm too knackered.

I don't want to have chemotherapy and poison my body. Yes I know it is the way to cure the cancer but would you want to feel sick, taste the chemicals in your mouth for days after, have to use mouthwash that makes you

1

urge, take so many tablets that you have to take more tablets to make you shit!

I don't want to choose the new bathroom tiles and know that I don't have the energy to help Trevor put them up.

I don't want to have a go at Trevor because I am frustrated at not being able to help with the house or garden. I know he understands because he tells me, but I want to do all I could before cancer.

I don't want family and friends to not talk about the chance that this might all go wrong and yes speak the words that "I might die". I am not stupid and I know that they must have all thought it but I seem to be the only one who dares to say it, this is not me giving up, this is me facing the possibilities because if you think that this cancer is going to win well maybe it should be your lights I am punching out!

But most of all I DON'T WANT TO LOSE MY HAIR.

I had my hair cut short yesterday which seems stupid as I write this, it's going to fall out in a few weeks anyway. "Get it cut short before it starts to fall out" everyone who seems to know anything about cancer suggests, well here's some news for you all, I DON'T WANT TO HAVE

IT CUT, in fact I don't want anyone to touch my hair because its fine as it is (even though I do like it now it has been cut but that's not the point!). My hair is the first outward sign to show to the world that I HAVE CANCER.

The one thing that I do want is my humour to keep going what ever happens. So on the hair front I am planning to turn into Gollum from Lord of the rings and audition for a part in the new West end play, my precious!

So how did I get to be in this state? Well you will have to wait until later in the morning for that as I now feel calmer and I am going back to bed. So thanks Kieran and goodnight.

This is how it all started.

August 10th 2006

Trevor and I are sat in bed watching the European Athletics on the TV at 9:30am and discussing whether to go blackberry picking or get my hair cut. As usual the Great Britain team is allowing others to win all the medals as we are such good losers. A hair cut must be a better option! I start to get out of bed and say to Trevor "it feels like I have just wet myself" I stand beside the bed and see blood pouring out of me. I run to the bathroom and still the blood flows.

Trevor grabs the phone to ring for an ambulance and in my usual calm way during an emergency I say "no just ring the doctor" so Trevor rings for an ambulance! I feel faint and lay on the floor, of course making sure that my bottom half is over the lino of the bathroom so it's easier to clear up later!

The male paramedics arrive and my dignity leaves (in fact I'm not sure that it has returned yet!). They sit me in a chair and wheel me to the ambulance while suggesting that I should move house to somewhere without steps and hills. I am then wired up to machines, needles inserted into my hand and a drip put up. Then off to the 'gynae' ward.

I lay in the ambulance joking with the paramedics but underneath I am scared. I try to make sense of what is happening to me but my humour kicks in again and I stop thinking and just go with the here and now.

There are several insights that I have had during this time the first being that you should not get admitted to hospital just after the 1st of August as this is when the new doctors start each year. And yes I got one who was able to treat me to my very own 'carry on' moment.

With me lying on a very hard trolley the doctor decides to perform an internal examination. Just what you need after you have just auditioned for the latest give blood campaign. So feet together, knees apart, up with the speculum, focus the light, he's going in. The doctor then looks up and around, moves the light, moves around again and announces that he can't see my cervix. Has it fallen out? Surely it can't be that far up inside, maybe I left it at home on the bathroom floor! The nurse to the rescue, "I'll have a look" she says and then the slow motion begins. She bends over to have a look and so does the doctor, unfortunately they are both looking at my nether regions and yes the inevitable happens. They smack heads with a loud thud and reel back, hands on foreheads seeing stars.

I can see the headlines. Doctor and nurse knocked out on floor, patient left on trolley, feet together, and knees apart!

I am wheeled off to a single room and at last allowed to get into a proper bed. Doctors are still coming in and asking questions which have already been asked by the doctor who was in two minutes ago. I am not allowed out of bed which is the time you really need to go to the toilet. I balance my bum on the bed pan and wonder whether I am weeing into the pan or is it going over the bed? What a relief when the pan is removed and I lay down in a dry bed. Next the bed bath to clean me up. It's a good job my dignity left when it did! You cannot believe how good this wash is, I feel clean again and the smell of dried blood has gone.

I'm sat talking to Trevor when the door to my room opens and the doctor asks if he can see me alone. Trevor leaves and the doctor sits on the chair beside my bed. He says that one of the blood tests has come back with an abnormal level (of what he does not say), he asked if there is any chance that I could be pregnant, well actually he went around the houses to ask the question as he was already aware that Trevor has had a vasectomy. Being the kind person I am I had already worked out what he was going go ask and decided that he needed to practice asking difficult questions, so I opted not to help him out! I informed him that I will either be suing a surgeon or this was the Immaculate Conception.

The doctor tells me he thinks I have had a miscarriage and that it is not unheard of for vasectomies to go wrong. I'm stunned. He asked if I have any questions, what does he expect me to ask!

The doctor leaves the room and Nurse Bridget returns. I tell her what the doctor has said and she says she knows and am I alright with that. I say "I only wanted to go blackberry picking"

Trevor comes back into the room and I tell him what the doctor has said. He's stunned!

I am visited by more doctors who continue to ask the same questions and I am told I will have an ultrasound to see what is going on inside me.

The rest of the day just seems to merge into one. My children arrive to see me, my youngest daughter Vicky brings me some clothes she has brought from my house. She has also cleaned up some of the blood and is a little shocked at the amount of blood I lost.

I am very tired, in fact I would go so far as to say knackered. Also I am very scared because as far as I am aware losing that amount of blood for no apparent reason is not normal. As usual I do not show how scared I am but use my humour to mask this.

The scan is going to be tomorrow which seems a long time away when you are scared of what they might find but neither Trevor or I would dare mention the 'C' word even though I am sure he is thinking it and I'm sure I am.

11ᵗʰ *August 2006*

The morning starts with being woken to have my obs taken. Why do they wake you up so early and then tell me I need to rest and not get out of bed! More blood tests, more doctors and more bed pans. Then I am allowed to walk to the toilet, it's amazing how little things become important to you. The walking to the toilet does not last long as when you are about to have an ultrasound you need to drink litres of water and not use the toilet. Eventually the call comes for me to go for my ultrasound scan. I walk over with Trevor and a nurse, desperate for a wee. I hope they don't want me to wait long.

I feel very nervous lying on another hard bed, stomach covered in cold gel and the screen facing me. The scan reveals something in my womb which the nurse describes as 'not a normal pregnancy'. What this means I do not know. I am not sure that Trevor has heard this and I'm too scared to ask. The nurse then decides to perform an internal scan (lucky me!) and asks me to wait in the room opposite so she can set everything up. Although this gives me more time to think I am allowed to go to the toilet, what a relief.

The doctor arrives to speak to us and says she has looked at the scan pictures and there is something there but she is not sure what it is but it could be fibroids. I know about fibroids and I know they are not the 'c' word, so I hold onto that. She also says that there does not appear to be any more blood so I can go home for the weekend but must return at 9:00am on Monday morning. Its like being given time off for good behaviour!

The ultrasound nurse calls me in again and gets me to lie at the end of the bed. She then realises that the cold air fan is pointing directly towards my nether regions and turns the thermal blast off! I ask if she will turn the fan on to suck and get rid of what is inside but the Health Service do not run to fans which do this!

I am released at 4:30pm and on the way home make several telephone calls to family and friends telling them that I am home for the weekend.

After wandering around the house and garden like I have not been there for weeks I sit on the sofa to watch television. It's 6:30pm. Then I feel the blood start to pump again. Already the blood is showing through my jeans. I run to the bathroom again while Trevor phones for an ambulance and my eldest daughter Becky phones the Gynae ward.

This time the blood pumps faster. The paramedics arrive to find me sat on the toilet with only my top clothes on. They put several pads on me plus two pairs of pants and quickly walk me to the ambulance outside the house.

By the time I get to the ambulance there is blood flowing down my legs. The blood pressure machine will not work and they can't get a needle in my veins. Still the blood pumps. Then the ambulance begins to spin. I say to the paramedic 'I think I am going' I can feel myself drifting in and out of consciousness and I am very scared. I know I have lost a lot of blood and I am not sure that I will wake up again if I pass out. I feel so scared that any words of reassurance from them are not enough.

I look over to Trevor who is sat in the ambulance but can't really see his face. The paramedic calls the driver into the back and I know that it is not going well. She jumps in and tells me it is alright to faint. So I do. I go into a vivid dream which I cannot now remember. Then someone is saying to me "you're alright, you are in an ambulance, you fainted". My tongue feels sore like it has been bitten and I spit out a piece of tooth. I look over to Trevor again

as he strokes my head and says "it's alright".
That's one of those things that people say isn't
it? Of course I'm not alright. At least I can see
him clearly now.

The driver gets into the front of the ambulance
and the paramedic asks for blue lights. Not
a good sign. Much of the journey I do not
remember, which is sad because if you are
going to be blue lighted into hospital you
should be able to remember the experience.
Maybe they will take me for a ride when I'm
better so I can experience the ride to the full!

I have a drip going into my arm which is normal,
what is <u>not</u> normal is the way she is squeezing
the bag to get the fluids into me.

As I am moved out of the ambulance on the
trolley somehow my arm gets knocked and
out comes the drip which shoots water over
my right shoulder like a fountain, well I needed
a shower with all the blood about! I can see
how fast I am being pushed down the corridor
because the strip lights have joined and
become one long light.

Then I'm back on the gynae ward with the
nurse Bridget who said goodbye to me 2½
hours ago. The blood in still pumping.

Bridget takes my blood pressure and I ask what it is through the oxygen mask she says 'it's alright' which means it's not. Doctor Carlos arrives who is aged about 6 but I will let him off as he is good looking. Trevor and Becky are also in the room and I hear Becky say "its only attention seeking behaviour", this makes me smile because this is a normal comment for my family. I start to shake uncontrollably which Bridget reassuringly explains it is the shock my body is in. Then she asks someone to get a registrar down and I hear the doctor telling Trevor that I might need to go to theatre tonight. Yes please I think to myself, just sort me out now.

The blood finally stops. Bridget asks if it is ok to cut my pants off. I don't want to keep them on so this is fine. I watch as they are put into the bin with the pads. They are soaked with blood so I look the other way. Two nurses arrive to clean me up again, and then it's off to my side room again. I am told not to move off my bed so I immediately need a bed pan, Bed pan in place Trevor and Bridget say they will leave the room to allow me some dignity, I say there is no point because when you have got to go, you've got to go. If I needed proof that my dignity had gone I think this is it.

The registrar arrives and asks the same questions as have been asked before (are doctors trained in this? Do they have special meetings with each other to make sure they are all asking the same questions?) She informs me that I will be staying in hospital. I say that is good because I am not going home until I am sorted out. She also says that I can drink and eat what I want because I will not need an operation tonight. I order a Pimms as this is the healthy option because of the fruit you put in it. The registrar says if I go and get the drink I can have it. This is where the bed rest really is a pain in the arse!

Trevor leaves at 12:30am looking absolutely shattered. Still neither of us are mentioning the 'C' word.

14th August 2006

The doctor who was 7 years old just now! tells me that it has been decided that they will have a look inside me tomorrow which will involve making a small cut just below my belly button and putting a camera inside me. This procedure will also require me to have a general anaesthetic, well that's a relief! So today I rest, well I have little choice because bungee jumping and hang gliding are difficult when you are on bed rest.

I have lots of visitors which is great because it stops me from thinking about the 'C' word for a while.

15th August 2006

The morning of my operation and nil by mouth, so the diet starts here. Mr. West the surgeon enters my room at 9:00am and shakes my hand. He then says that he has passed my case onto another surgeon who will be visiting me very soon to talk about my operation, so it was nice to meet me and goodbye. Well that was short and sweet.

The door opens again and Mr. Rennison enters with a woman they both sit on my bed and I look at the badge which says Gail, gynae/ oncology specialist nurse. I can hear Mr. Rennison talking to me but I can't take in what he is saying. All I can see is the word oncology, I know this means cancer.

I refocus to hear that I am going to be having a hysterectomy because there is a growth in my womb. The hormone test also shows that this could be a rare form of cancer and if I was to ask him then there is a 1 in 5 chance that I have cancer. Well at least someone is saying the 'c' word. I will be having my womb and cervix taken out and do I want my ovaries removed as well. How the hell do I know! There is this badge starring at me saying YOU HAVE CANCER. Apparently I do not have to make my mind up immediately. Well that's unlikely because my mind is somewhere else at the moment. Mr. Rennison says he will be back about 12ish and leaves me with Gail.

She sits quietly beside me on my bed but I am unable to say how I feel instead I tell her that I am fine, which does not fool her or me.

She leaves to give me time to think. I ask the nurse if I can get my husband in because of the news I have just been given. Of course she replies then I realise that all the staff would already know the content of the conversation with Mr. Rennison.

I calmly walk outside to use my mobile to dial Trevor's number and as soon as he talks I burst into tears. I manage to tell him what is happening and through the tears ask him to come quick.

I cry my way back to my room and a nurse spots me and asks if I am alright, I say no. She sits with me while I cry. I don't seem to be able to make any sense of what is happening to me. I just cry.

Trevor arrives and for the first time we talk openly about the possibility that I could have cancer. He says that if there is a 1 in 5 chance I have cancer then there is a 4 in 5 chance that I do not.

We discuss what kind of operation I should have, which is difficult as I do not remember a 10th of what was said to me, so I ask for Gail to return.

Gail explains everything again and this time I hear most of it. I decide that while they are operating on me they might as well take everything. What do I need my reproductive system for and if there is a chance that my ovaries have cancer as well then I don't want another operation.

Mr. Rennison returns and I explain that I would like the full works which he says he thinks is the right choice. He leaves saying he will see me in theatre later. I hope not as I want to be asleep by then!

The anaesthetist arrives to check my breathing and asks if I want morphine or an epidural after the operation. I am no martyr so opt for the epidural. I am then weighed, measured and x-rayed, a full service. This also means to me that this is a major operation and the nerves begin.

At 12:00 1 shower ready for the main event and put on one of the lovely hospital gowns which is marked 'hospital property only'. Who would want to take one of these and where would they wear it? It's better not to dwell on this!

Trevor is still with me and the minutes start to roll by, then the hours roll by. The door opens at 9:30 pm and Mr. Rennison appears, not looking at his best. He explains that there have been some emergency operations and there were more to come. He acknowledges that my condition is serious but not life threatening. I look at how tired he looks and although I would prefer my operation to go ahead I would also prefer to have the right bits removed and I could not guarantee that in his state this would happen. He assures me that the operation will take place tomorrow lunchtime. I thank him for coming to tell me himself and he leaves.

I am so tired with the stress of the day that sleeping is not going to be a problem and I am also allowed to eat and drink until midnight. Don't get too excited at the last statement as all that is left on the ward at that time of night are sandwiches!

Trevor leaves and I settle down for the night.

16th August 2006

I get up and shower again ready for the main event part 2. Trevor arrives to be with me and at 11:00am the nurse brings in my pre-med with what she informs me are antibiotics and paracetamol. Where are the mind altering drugs that send you into the dream world? Apparently they do not use them anymore, sadists!

The ward phone rings at 12:00 to ask for me to go to theatre, but do they take me on my bed or in a wheelchair? No I have to walk and carry my own pillow! What is the NHS coming to?

As I am about to the leave the ward there is a call for Trevor. It's our friends Jen and Rob who will be in the café in 5 minutes to sit with Trevor. This is a great relief to me that someone will be with him during my operation. I kiss him goodbye at the lifts and go into the theatre corridor with the nurse.

Suddenly everything seems very serious and I feel very nervous. I am greeted by the anaesthetist and guided into the room next to the operating theatre. I can hear music coming from the theatre, I wonder what they are playing is it 'the first cut is the deepest'?!

The anaesthetist asks me to sit on the side of the bed and hold my head over my pillow so he can start the epidural. He numbs my back with local anaesthetic which stings. Then he inserts a long needle into my back which I wish I had not looked at. The room starts to spin so I tell the nurse I feel faint. On with the oxygen mask and they have not even started to operate yet. This is not a good start. Why didn't you knock me out first I ask? Because it is better if you are awake. I'm not sure about that one!

I am laid down on the trolley and within minutes I can feel my eyes closing. "Nikki it's all over and you are in the recovery room". It feels like I have been asleep for 3 seconds but the clock indicates 2 ½ hours. How does that work? Maybe I can do time travel after all!

Back on the ward I am wheeled into the side room but the bed is facing a different way. Did they move the room and all the electrics around to fool me? No this is a different room! They have moved me to the other end of the ward. Did I misbehave? No they are shutting one end of the ward; it must have been something I said! Anyway in my room are Trevor, Vicky and my dad and a balloon saying get well soon from Jen and Rob. But where is my TV aerial I ask Trevor. He laughs and says that only I would notice that after an operation. I insist that he goes to get it, so he does. Vicky leaves and I ask her to give her dog a kiss from me! I think that maybe the anaesthetic has worked! Everyone leaves me to sleep, well when I say sleep that is in between being woken up to have my obs done, frequently!

17th August 2006

I wake to realise that I am wired for sound! I have a drip in my arm, an epidural in my back, a drain tube in my stomach and a catheter up my **!!. But there is no pain. I spoke to soon. It's bed bath time and lucky me I get to sit in the chair which is a little difficult when you can't feel your feet and they seem to have independent motion! With the aid of two nurses I manage the task. I collapse back into bed after 5 minutes and I am exhausted.

Next few days 2006
I must admit that the next few days become a bit of a blur with the following highlights....

My friend Jane arrives with a card that says 'welcome to the uterus free club' she also informs me that I am now a woman of a certain age and presents me with a copy of the People's Friend magazine. She produces a bag of tomatoes because as she says "everyone brings grapes".

My friend Colleen arrives with a card that says 'if you did not want to cook for me we could have eaten at Ikea, she gives me a packet of muesli and 4 tins of fish.

My friend Jen arrives and asks me what kind of operation I had was it a full English or just a continental? I tell her it was a full English.

With friends like these who needs enemies?

These friends are also looking after Trevor, as are my family. Trevor needs support as well and I am not able to do this at present. The only thing is that they are all asking him the same questions which he is becoming a bit paranoid about. He tells me they are all asking if he has taken his tablets and has he eaten!

I need to mention the hospital food at this point as all my visitors ask how it is. Well they asked. You would think that if someone is unwell they would make the food appetising, but I don't think that Jamie Oliver has been to the hospital kitchens. The menu includes: cheese and potato bake, shepherds pie and chips all at the same time. Why do you need chips when there is already potato in the other dishes? Sunday lunch is a real treat, brown cardboard, shredded green paper and elasticated Yorkshire puddings known in another form as roast beef with cabbage and Yorkshire puds! The gravy was good. Deserts featured banana less banana cake. I would like to point out that the fresh fruit and sandwiches appeared very popular, not sure why!

Because I am diabetic I don't get to wear those lovely white stockings, no I get to wear calf socks which explode with a puff of air every minute or so. The machine that makes them work is hooked on the end of my bed which makes the bed continually vibrate. I have to be strapped into them as I am unable to bend. I have one of my funny moments when Bridget comes to strap me in one night, switches the machine on and then says I look hot, and do I have too many clothes on?. I reply to her saying. Dear matron, the nurse strapped me to the bed, made it vibrate knowing that I cannot have sex for six weeks and then asked me if I wanted to take my clothes off'.

I am visited by the physiotherapist who goes through the do's and don'ts booklet. Apparently I can work up to doing housework like ironing; I have been personally working up to ironing for 45 years and feel I have some way to go. 'I will not have a problem with stairs when I get home'. I tell her I will because we live in a bungalow and don't have any! I will get Trevor to put some in before I get home. I can't have sex for 6 weeks, the way I feel at the moment 6 months would be too soon.

I have started to have hot flushes which I am told is the beginning of the menopause caused by the hysterectomy. Well that's nice! So within just over a week I have had two haemorrages, a hysterectomy, started the change and I have possibly got cancer. Well I can't say life is boring!

One night I wake up and burst into tears. I feel like I am on a rollercoaster with no end to the track. I keep thinking to myself that I am intelligent woman (trust me on this!) so why can't I make sense of what is happening to me. I know all the events that have happened but cannot fit them together in my head. I call a nurse who sits with me for a while, calms me down and I drift back to sleep.

The morning arrives with Gail who has been told of my tears. I explain to her that I feel very confused not only by the events that have happened but also I can't process them. In her usual calm way which I find very reassuring she explains that the experience I have had is similar to being in a coma where you lose track of time. She goes and gets my hospital notes and reads through them with me. I begin to understand that the abnormal level in my blood is a hormone which is linked to pregnancy. The normal level for a woman is between 0-4, my level before the hysterectomy was 117,000. A little on the high side! Seeing the notes as well as hearing them makes the pieces of the past few days fit again. This immediately calms me.

Then the humour starts again. I ask if the all this is possibly linked to the triplets that I gave birth to in the pantomime I was in, in February? She seems to think this is unlikely but makes a mental note that Trevor and I spent two nights in a hotel during a recent house move because our buyer failed to pay his money on time! I am not sure what she thinks we did during those nights (well I do but I am not saying!).

Gail explains that it will take ten days to two weeks for the results of the histology to come back. There is nothing I can do during this time but that will not stop me thinking about the results.

21st August 2006

The ward seems very quiet today and all the nurses are working just at one end. I wander down for lunch to find that I am one of four patients left. Over lunch I realise that the rest of the patients are all leaving today and I will be the only person on a forty one bed ward. Who needs private medical care when you have your own team of doctors, nurses and ancillary staff! I am assured by staff that more patients will be coming in later.

During the afternoon visiting a nurses head keeps appearing at my door and asking if I am alright. The poor nurses have to sit in their room because I don't need any care at present. I offer to make an illness up but they decline. You just can't help some people.

22nd August 2006

Staples out today. I decide not to count them as they come out for fear of being included in the Guinness book of records for the most ever staples in a stomach.

During my time in hospital I have used a visualisation of a beach to manage my feelings when medical interventions were being performed on me. So I go and sit on my imaginary piece of drift wood and watch the waves wash in while the nurse unstapled me. All is well, I do not explode open, what a relief.

I am told by the doctor that I can go home and suddenly I feel scared. I have been in the safety of the hospital for twelve days and the last time I went home was a disaster. I now have to go home again without any nurses or doctors as a safety net. Trevor arrives to take me home and I say my goodbyes. I arrive home and feel very unsettled. I know I can phone the ward if there are any problems but that does not seem enough. It takes about two hours for me to settle down and begin to relax. I am starting to believe that I will be alright. I fall into bed exhausted by recent events and drift off to sleep.

23rd August 2006

Well I spoke too soon! The bottom of my wound is leaking and it is beginning to sting. So Trevor phones the ward and back in we go. I feel safe back on the ward but know that I am not staying the night. After a dressing and antibiotics I am on my way home again.

I have noticed that when I feel tired it's like a wave of sleepiness engulfs me and I have no choice but to lay down and sleep. It's a strange feeling but not one that I can fight, so I learn to give into it and obey.

24th August 2006

Jen takes me to hospital today to have my dressing changed and I tell her that I have had a phone call from the hospital asking me to come to the results clinic on Tuesday 29th. I say calmly that I am expecting to hear that I could have cancer as this is what I have been told is the possibility.

As the day passes at home I feel myself getting low, so I go to bed early in the evening hoping the feeling will go away. Trevor is finding it difficult to manage his own feelings about having to wait for the result of the histology. He wants me to phone Gail tomorrow and demand answers.

This is too much pressure for me as I have been trying to put such thoughts out of my mind. In fact just at the moment I would rather not know. Then the tears start which soon turn to sobbing uncontrollably and I feel alone and lost. Whatever Trevor says does not calm me and finally he has run out of things to say, plus I do not want to talk to him. Trevor picks up the phone and rings Jen. She arrives and says "you out of bed" pointing to me and "you make the tea" looking at Trevor. I crawl out of bed into the front room and tell her what has happened. I am convinced in my own mind that I have cancer and I do not want to die.

Jen eventually calms me down, sends me back to bed, and tucks me in for the night. Then returns home. I am now talking to Trevor and can understand a bit more how he feels. Thankfully that feeling is mutual so sleep comes soon.

The weekend 2006

The weekend is spent partly talking about what might be and partly avoiding the subject. The time seems to drag and the closer it gets to Tuesday the more the tension rises.

29th August 2006

The day of the result clinic finally arrives and we get to the hospital in plenty of time. I am unable to sit for too long as the toilet keeps calling me.

I notice Gail in the distance and feel like I am staring at her. I am watching her face in case she looks at me and gives something away. The more I try not to look at her the stronger the urge to watch her grows. She sees me and says not long now, but gives nothing away.

Mr. Rennison is on holiday, so I will be seeing another surgeon and Gail today. At last Gail calls my name, and Trevor and I follow her into the consulting room. The surgeon, Mr. Achenson tells me that as they thought unfortunately I do have a rare form of cancer. What he says next I do not know as my mind has stopped on "I have cancer" and yes my humour kicks in and I reply "well I needed a hair cut anyway". Apparently this is not a normal thing to say at this time! He goes on to tell me it is called Chorio something or other but I just want to leave the room. I mention that the wound is still leaking so he asks to take a look and at last I get the chance to leave. I go into the side room, closely followed by Gail. I sit on the bed and don't know where to put myself. I ask her the question that has been going around in my head, "am I going to live," she replies "I can't answer that". Of course she can't but it's what I want to know.

After the examination I return to the consulting room and notice a door on the other side of the room which says vacant. I want to go through that door and change the sign to say engaged and stay there by myself.

I pull myself together enough to ask for some written information on my condition so at least I can refer to it when I feel able to. I also manage to take onboard that the cancer is so rare that I will be referred to Charing Cross hospital in London as this is the centre that treats it in this country. I am also being referred for a scan of my head, chest and pelvis to see if the cancer has spread.

Mr. Achenson apologises for not giving me the news I wanted to hear and I am off at the speed of light, out the door towards the lifts being closely followed by Trevor and Gail. She is telling him she will ring in a few days, I can see her watching me but I am in the lift already and am not going to hang around for anyone.

In the car outside I flip back into my outer calmness. I agree to go and see my dad and step mum. Inside I feel devastated. I have questions flying around my head which includes the big question, "am I going to die?" How long do I have to live?" The questions are so horrible that I am afraid to put them into spoken words.

We arrive at my dad and step mums' house I tell them calmly that I have cancer but don't show how I am feeling inside because I don't think I know myself. I ask Trevor to speak to our children as I don't feel able to talk to them yet. I know if I do I will cry, and that's not what they need at the moment.

The rest of the day is a daze. I try to get my head around what is happening. It feels like the roller coaster has started again and I can't see the station.

Trevor phones our new doctor as we have just moved and I have not met him yet. I get an appointment that afternoon which can't come too soon.

I immediately feel relaxed with Dr Sweeney as he tells me to call him Kieran (I still blame him for this which is now beginning to be a book!) I suggest that I stay on one of my tablets as 'I'm ill you know' he tells me he is the doctor and will be the judge of that. I have got a doctor with a sense of humour which is just what I need. I ask for a certificate, and he replies "you want time off work?" How long?" So I tell him he is the doctor so he can be the judge of that! We both laugh and I know I will be able to talk to him when things get tough, and I'm sure they will.

I am told to keep in touch with him and that the staff at the surgery are there to work for me. I am also invited to call in or ring whenever I need to, even if it's only to talk.

I return home feeling reassured that the medical care will be there for me when I need it, and also the emotional support which I am sure I will need.

Another next few days 2006

I try to continue on with my life while waiting for a scan appointment and a letter to be admitted to Charing Cross. By sheer coincidence I have to call an ambulance for a family member and the paramedic who arrives is the same one who picked me up on the second bleed. She recognises me and says that the ambulance looked like the 'chain saw massacre' after I had left it. This is too much information, but I do find it funny.

I have a phone call from Gail telling me that Charing cross hospital will be expecting me as an inpatient as of 11th September. I had got it into my head that I was just going for the day but I could be there for a week plus. I am told that there will be a lot of waiting about during the week for tests, but hopefully by the end of the week I will know what kind of treatment I will need. Well I can't complain about having to wait around for the NHS to do something. The problem is every time another appointment is made the rollercoaster starts again, and I am not telling anyone how I feel about the ride.

6th September 2006

Scan day and I have made a CD to be played during the time in the scanner. Of course I choose music for the moment! To start I have 'don't stop me now, I'm having such a good time, I'm having a ball'. Followed by 'I want to break free'. Trevor has told me that 'another one bites the dust' may not be appropriate, but it makes me laugh!

I dress in another of those designer hospital gowns with rear access. I am led into the scanning room. I offer my CD to be told they do not play them on a CT scan, only during an MRI scan. But I am just as nervous whatever kind of scan it is so why don't they?

I lay on the bed and am asked if I could be pregnant. I know by this that they have not read my notes, so ask what the chances are considering that I had a hysterectomy 3 weeks ago. She smiles at me and then continues to position me ready for the scan.

I am told be breathe in, then hold my breath, then breathe out. As the scanner moves up and down my body I wonder what it is finding and what the radiologist is seeing. Has the cancer spread? I have read that it could be in my vagina, lungs or brain. I wonder where it is, and then start to sing the songs on my CD in my head.

The scan is soon over and I don't even try to ask if they have found anything knowing that they cannot tell me.

8th September 2006

I have been asked to carry the scan pictures to Charing Cross to ensure that they get there on time. This means that they spend the weekend burning a hole in my dining room table. I am not tempted to look as I don't want to see just in case the cancer has spread, also I am not sure which way up they should be!

11 September 2006

We have asked my brother, (Simon) to take us to Charing Cross as I feel Trevor may be a little too stressed to drive around London. So up at the crack of dawn and off we go. Trevor feels unable to eat breakfast before we leave which he regrets later after the service station breakfast!

We arrive at clinic 8 Charing Cross in good time and I have blood taken. The phlebotomist then asks for a sample of Trevor's blood. This stuns me, but it's good to share these things. Trevor goes and gives blood and is told it is for research.

Simon has gone off to find Trevor's' bed and breakfast. He returns and asks the address again, as the one Trevor has given him is an estate agent. After several minutes and some lateral thinking Simon goes to explore again. He finds the B & B in the other direction, in a different road.

Then my name is called and Professor Seckl introduces himself and helps Trevor and I to wheel the suitcases into the consulting room. We are introduced to Linda, who is my new specialist nurse and two doctors. I pass over the scan pictures and Professor Seckl looks at them. He says that he cannot see any spread of the cancer on them, but will get them checked to be sure. In my nervousness I tell the professor that I drink six litres of alcohol a week. The young doctor is suddenly awake, and Trevor quickly comes to my rescue and reminds me it should be units and that I probably only drink three to four <u>units</u> a week. That's my street cred gone!

Professor Seckl says he will come and see me later and Linda directs us with what has become one of her legendry map drawings! So we follow the wall signs and find our way to 6 south ward.

Although Gail has told me I would be going onto a cancer ward, a shock to the system would be an understatement! There is cancer staring me in the face, and I want to be anywhere but here.

I realise that I have nowhere near come to terms with my cancer.

Trevor is with me on the ward when Professor Seckl arrives and says that they have not found any trace of the cancer spreading, but that I do have a pool of some liquid just under my scar, which they will aspirate tomorrow. He also tells me that they will start my Chemotherapy at the end of the week. I agree with the plan, not really thinking about the implications for me.

After the professor has left I do start to think. I thought I was only coming up for tests. And now I am on a cancer ward, and going to be starting Chemo this week. I feel like I am in shock and I'm not sure if I had been told any of this before I would have been able to take it on board.

That night after Trevor has left to go to his B&B I lie awake wondering what is happening to me, and the rollercoaster starts again. I manage to calm myself down enough to sleep for a few hours.

12th September 2006

I am woken by the person in the next bed throwing up. This is becoming a nightmare! Is this what I will go through during my Chemo?

I go to find a nurse to talk to. By the time I find one I am in tears, feeling a long way from home and isolated. She suggests that I get Trevor in as it is now 9:00am. I phone him in tears, and he says he is on his way.

He gently holds me and calms me down. Now two of the people on the ward are throwing up. I need someone to give me information about Chemo, as what I don't know my imagination tends to make up, therefore the more info I have the better. The nurse says she will get Linda to come and see me, so I stop my mind working overtime and have a shower.

The porter arrives to take me down to x-ray for my aspiration. Trevor is allowed to accompany me, which is a great relief as I haven't got a clue what they are going to do to me. I know it has been explained to me by Linda but my head was somewhere else yesterday!

I am wheeled down on my bed which feels bizarre as I am perfectly able to walk. But who am I to argue? My bed is pushed into an x-ray room next to the ultrasound machine. The doctor puts some cold gel over my stomach (I have been here before!), he says that there is not much liquid there now but it would be better to get it out. I am then injected with local anaesthetic into my stomach, which stings and then quickly goes numb. It is very difficult to look anywhere else but towards the large needle being pushed into my stomach! I try to turn my head the other way but my neck muscles don't seem to be working. The doctor is looking at the ultrasound screen while moving the syringe in my stomach; it feels like I am a remote control. Then to finish me off he pulls the fluid out of my stomach through the syringe. Well at least I have not given birth to the alien!

I am returned to the ward and in the afternoon Linda comes to talk to us about chemotherapy. She has lots of printed information which I can read when she has gone. She slowly talks us through all the literature, and leaves us to look at it while she is still on the ward. Now I have information I can stop the rollercoaster, as I feel more in control.

Linda passes the bottom of my bed and I ask if I can talk to her. I ask if there is a separate room to have my chemo in. She looks surprised and tells me that you have it on the ward. I point out to her that in the information she has given me it says 'you can have sex during treatment;' well I'm not too keen on having sex in a four bed ward! Apparently no one has spotted this before; well they haven't met me before! She tells me that this is the NHS and to just pull the curtains around!

I read some more of the information, which tells me that 1 in 50,000 women get this kind of cancer. So I am the chosen one! Next time I'm the chosen one it had better be the lottery!

I go outside the hospital to phone everyone to let them know that I am starting chemo tomorrow. I mention to Jane that I will lose my hair, and she tells me to think of what I will save on waxing! She's such a gem!

I also phone Colleen and tell her the same information as Jane. Colleen asks if she can sign my head when I am bald. She says that if I had broken my arm then she would sign the plaster, so it is only right that she should sign my head. I do worry about my friends!

I later find out that you can use your mobile in the hospital so I won't be going out into the cold again. I wondered why everyone had there mobiles by their beds!

13 September 2006

The delights of chemotherapy today. I know, my life just gets better! I have a cannula put in the back of my hand and although I may seem calm outside I am terrified inside.

The thought of all those chemicals going into my body is almost too much to take, but I know this is the only possibility to get rid of the cancer; so my fight begins.

I have a metal taste in my mouth and feel a little bit sick, but apart from that I hope that all my chemo's will be this easy. I am no fool though and realise that there is an accumulative effect with chemo, so they won't all be this easy.

14 September 2006

My brother arrives to take us home. Unfortunately the pharmacy has not sent my tablets up yet, so after another hour's wait we get to leave. I sit in the back of the car feeling sorry for myself but glad to be going home. We stop at Cheveley services for a comfort stop (posh hey!) It is not long after we have started on our way again that I fall asleep. I wake a few miles from my house and have slept for about three hours. I may have been a little tired!

I fall into bed exhausted but I don't care. I am in my own bed, with my own duvet and pillow and that's where I am staying.

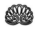

Another few days 2006 part 2

I sleep most of the days but don't feel too bad. I'm sure I should feel and look worse than I do but hey I've got to feel well at some points.

I don't want you to think that I am being left to rest, no; I have blood tests to attend, so the stabbing continues.

19th September 2006

Charing Cross today, first to see another consultant in clinic 8 then up to day case to have chemo. We leave at 7:00am and drive up the M5 where the mist is floating low in the fields. I am aware that I notice details like this more now. The thought of why I look at details more briefly enters my head then my humour clicks in, and I turn to Trevor and say 'If I did not have cancer we would not have seen this'.

We have borrowed my daughters Sat Nav to stop the loud discussion which usually takes place as to whether I point right or left (saying right or left takes me a while to work out which is which) and whether Trevor turned left or right. I programme it in the service station but I am not sure what number Charing Cross hospital is in Fulham Palace Road, so I put in 30 which with my luck will be the vets! We did manage to find the hospital alright

The consultant calls me in and asks how I am. He does not seem to make eye contact and sits behind a desk. This puts a barrier between us, and I know he is a good doctor but I communicate better with people who talk to me directly and do not put obstacles in the way of language. I want to say to him I am a human being with cancer not a cancer with human being, but I am too scared, so I don't.

He says I can go up to 6 west (day case) to have my chemo, so off I go.

Trevor and I wait for five hours for the chemo; this happens after Trevor talks to a sister and explains that we have a long journey back home.

We get to leave at 5:40pm and hit the London traffic. I manage to sit still until Cheveley services and ask Trevor to stop. On returning to the car I switch on the Sat Nav and change the voice to 'Tim'. He guides us to the roundabout outside the services and tells us to turn around when possible, so we do. The road leads us back to the services. We perform this manoeuvre three times and eventually follow the sign that says M4 Oxford. I know we don't want to go to Oxford, but we also don't want to spend the rest of the night in the service station! It turns out that the M4 west is also this way and we are off again.

Trevor demands that I turn the 'Jane' voice back on the Sat Nav as 'Tim' does not know what he is saying!

24ᵗʰ September 2006

I wake to find that I am wet at the bottom of the hysterectomy wound. As I feel down with my finger it disappears into a hole. So it's off the hospital again. The doctor looks at the hole and calls it a sinus. I thought they were in your nose, maybe it's slipped! The doctor says that is will heal alright and sends me home.

Later that day I don't feel very happy with what the doctor has said so talk to a friend who is a retired doctor. She suggests that I may need the sinus packing and to go to my surgery in the morning.

25ᵗʰ *September 2006*

I see the nurse at the doctor's surgery who confirms that I do need the sinus hole packed with seaweed. Does this mean a trip to the beach? No it comes in strip form and turns to gel when it gets wet. So I am patched back together, put on more antibiotics and look forward to being redressed every two days.

27ᵗʰ *September 2006*

Off to Charing Cross today for chemo so the alarm wakes us up at 6:30am. We manage to get on the road by 7:15 and I programme the Sat Nav with Jane's voice, as Trevor thinks Tim is useless after his last attempt to navigate us out of Cheveley services.

We arrive at the hospital at noon and yes the bed is not ready! So we escape from the ward and go for a walk around Hammersmith Broadway. Trevor got his glasses fixed that he had somehow managed to break on the journey up, so the time was not wasted!

After lunch we return to the ward and wait a further two hours for a bed. The doctor looks at the sinus hole and goes to phone the professor. At 5:00pm it is decided that my chemo would be put off for one week to allow some healing to take place. The doctor wants to also change my antibiotics.

I am asked if I want to stay the night in hospital. I don't think so, I want to go home.

When you are on chemo you can smell the chemicals as you walk up to the ward and the last thing I want to do is spend a night listening to people being sick and having my nose blocked by the smell. So off we go home.

Of course there is a traffic jam which holds us up for an hour and we eventually get home at 11:45pm.

28ᵗʰ September 2006

I wake up with a head cold and remember reading in one of the many information packs that I have been given that I am supposed to tell someone if I have an infection. So I ring Charing Cross, to be told to go to my nearest A & E department. A question now poses itself in my head, why do I get sent to a place where there is a risk of infection if I have an infection? I don't ponder this very long as life is too short!

So off to the hospital Trevor and I go. It is 8.05am and this was a day when I had no medical appointments planned, well I don't want to break my routine!

I feel stupid going to a hospital for a cold but as I have been told to go this makes it okay. I see the triage nurse who takes the same details as I know the doctor will ask and then sit in the waiting room for 1 ½ hours. During this time I amuse myself people watching.

One hankie on head, maybe his brain is going to fall out, a mother with her child who is called Jack. This I know because she used it so many times while trying to keep him in the waiting room and a woman holding her right elbow and wincing in pain that is until she uses it to open the toilet door! So toilet doors must have wonderful healing powers not yet known to the NHS.

'Nicola Coombs' comes the voice from the door and in I go. I explain that I am on chemo and have woken up with a head cold. After various breathing in and out, pushing in the stomach, instruments inserted into ears and mouth the doctor tells me I have a cold. The wonders of modern science are a joy to behold. Go home and rest is the advice. Well if I remember rightly that's what I was doing two hours ago. Is it me?

30ᵗʰ September 2006

My scalp starts to feel sore and tender to the touch. My hair has already thinned but now when I run my fingers thought my hair I bring out more than one strand. It will not be long before I have to wear my head scarf. I still don't want my hair to fall out so try not to think about what I will look like. The problem is the more you try not to think about something the more the thoughts engulf you. I feel low in the evening. There does not appear to be any reason why, well apart from having cancer that is.

1ˢᵗ October 2006

The district nurse is coming to redo my dressing this morning so I can shower. I remove the dressing not wanting to look in fact it makes me feel sick thinking about having a hole in me and it is becoming sore. I peel back the sticky outside and remove a few more of my pubic hairs; well they will be gone soon anyway.

My scalp is still sore, my hair needs washing but I don't want to touch it. I get in the shower and start washing my hair. This time as I rub my hair there is definitely not as much hair as before. I towel dry it gently in he vain hope that it will stay in longer.

4ᵗʰ October 2006

Off to Charing Cross with our usual early morning start. This time we stop at Membury services, which is another service station to tick off the list. We arrive in good time at the ward and the bed is not free which means that I am spared the ward lunch and head rapidly towards the hospital restaurant.

Returning to the ward I catch up with Peter the wig man and my new friend Nina, my wig. She's a little mouse coloured number. I tried on four different wigs but you just know when you have the right one and Nina is it. I have still not got my head around losing my hair (pardon the pun!), so I go with the flow of the moment and just agree with what I am being told about the aftercare of Nina. She needs to be washed with baby shampoo and then hung over a large bottle to dry. I'm not sure what she eats but as long as she does not have a nappy to be changed I'm happy.

I got a bed at 3:30pm. I am visited by the usual doctor who tells me that the professor and Linda will be up to see me. He also says that they need to do another blood test and my white cell count is low. This had better not be another wasted journey!

The professor and Linda arrive to tell me that I do have choriocarcinoma and my Beta HCG count is now 37. It seems a bit weird to be celebrating that I have choriocarcinoma but this type of cancer is very curable, so celebrate we do.

It has been pointed out to me that although I have mentioned that my cancer is called Choriocarcinoma I have not explained exactly what it is. So here goes in laywoman's terms. Choriocarcinoma is when a piece of placenta is left in the womb after the birth of a child. The piece of placenta is taken into the lining of the womb and can remain there for years. Unfortunately mine became cancerous. The information I have gathered from various medical professionals has told me that my cancer is unusual because it has remained in my body for so long, as my children are 20 and 25 years old. There again, as you may have come to realise there is nothing usual about me!

The professor decides that because I am responding so well to the chemo that it should go ahead despite my hole. In his words 'we should crack on and bite the bullet'. I suggest that I should crack on and he can bite the bullet. He agrees as long as the bullet does not explode!

My blood test comes back with an improvement so chemo goes ahead.

October 5ᵗʰ 2006

Chemo finishes at 1:00pm and then there is the usual wait for the pharmacy to send the drugs I need to the ward. Why they cannot sort the tablets the day before I don't know but it is probably someone's job to make sure that you stay longer in the hospital!

We leave at 2:00pm and I am asleep before we leave the outskirts of London. I wake again at Taunton which gives us the opportunity of visiting Taunton Deane Services. Another service station off the list.

We arrive home at 6:00pm and I fall into bed. There is one tablet after chemo that has to be taken at precise times, twelve hours apart so 7:30pm and 7:30am. I take the evening tablet and two hours later I am throwing up.

Trevor phones Charing Cross who suggests I come in for an injection. He explains that we are 3 ½ hours away so we contact the local duty doctor who arrives at my house at 12:30am stabs me in the bottom with a needle to stop me being sick and leaves. My life is just so exciting.

The injection works thank goodness as being up acid flavoured sick is not my favourite pastime. I eventually get to sleep about 1:30.

October 6th 2006

9:10 and my first medical intervention of the day. An appointment with Melissa at the doctors for a blood test. I return home and crawl back into bed still feeling a little sick and very sorry for myself. This is the worst effects of the chemo so far. I know that I will not be out of bed again today I just lay in a daze of tiredness and self pity.

When will this all end? How much longer will I have to go through this? I just want my life back. I remember that I should feel better in a day or two and try to hold onto that thought. Eating is beyond me but I do have something to look forward to. The district nurse is coming in the afternoon to give me an injection called

GCSF to boost my white blood cells. Then I will have the side effects of flu like symptoms to look forward to!

I feel that I should tell you what a typical week looks for me at the moment, so here goes: Monday - sinus dressing, Tuesday - blood tests, Wednesday - chemo, Thursday – dressing am. Injection pm, Friday – blood tests am. Injection pm, Saturday – dressing and injection pm. Sunday – injection. What a busy person I am! Seriously there are days when I wish I could be left alone and have some kind of normal life. I would love to have just a few days away, walking on a quiet beach, and miles from anywhere. Maybe in the future!

October 9ᵗʰ 2006

My hair has been falling out for some weeks now but I have not managed to gather the courage to have it cut off. Well this morning I wake up with a mouth full of hair. That is enough to make me sort my hair out.

I go to my hairdresser and ask for my hair to be cut off. Another hairdresser who does not know me says 'you don't want your hair all cut off really do you'. I resist telling her across the shop and choose to say nothing.

My hairdresser takes me to the back of the shop and cuts either side of my hair off. Then asks me if I want to keep the Mohican. This makes me laugh which is just what I need. I decline so she cuts my hair to a grade one all over. I ask if she could save some of the hair as I need some in another place that is also losing its hair!

I have taken Nina, my wig with me and she cuts it to suit my head shape. I leave with Nina and walk towards the car where Trevor is. I am feeling that everyone knows I have a wig on. I'm sure I will get use to her in time.

I realise at lunchtime that my scalp does not hurt anymore. If I knew that this would happen I would have had my hair cut sooner as even laying my head on the pillow at night hurt.

I have had a few problems with Nina since she came into my life as she has been living on a bottle filled with gin and blackcurrants which is maturing for Christmas. I think she might have been drinking the contents and I swear in the mornings she is hanging sideways over the bottle.

My family and friends now go into overdrive with the humour of the hair cut by which I mean comments like: "I should have gone to scarf savers," Why don't you open a shop called scarves r us" and my favourite by Trevor that I am 'baldly going where no one has been before'.

Well it makes me laugh!

October 10ᵗʰ 2006

It's the middle of the night and I have been awake since the early hours coughing. The thrush is causing the back of my throat to glue together; well that's what it feels like! I leave the marital bed and decamp to the sofa. The telly has some interesting programmes on at this time of night. I now know how to manufacture a space satellite and how to mine gold in North America.

The morning brings the usual round of telephone calls including explaining that I am unable to send the form requested by Exeter City Council within five days. As the Department of Work and pensions has not sent me the form yet. Why can't government departments speak to each other I'm ill you know and don't need to sort them out as well.

We visit my dad and step mum who are staying in a local hotel. I order the seafood platter for lunch it arrives with bread rolls and salad. I manage to eat all the seafood but it is too painful with the thrush to eat anything else so although I am still hungry I leave the food.

I suggest that we have a game of snooker. Trevor plays first, next my dad then it's my turn. I bend down over the table to line up the cue with the ball but Nina has other ideas. Bending my head back causes my wig to rise up the back of my head and start to come off. I begin to laugh, pull of the wig and revert to wearing a scarf. Do they make sports wigs I wonder?

October 11ᵗʰ 2006

One of my chemo's can now to be undertaken in Exeter which is going to make life a bit easier. I feel at home at Cherrybrook day case unit which I think has got a lot to do with the fact that it is a hospital that I am familiar with and it is not as busy as Charing Cross. My appointment is at 12:30 and although we have to wait for the chemo to arrive at the unit there is no pressure to get on the road as the journey takes 15 minutes not 4 hours.

The chemo goes well and I am home by 5:00pm. I wish that all my chemo's could be done at Cherrybrook but this is not possible, and anyway Charing Cross would miss me!

October 12ᵗʰ 2006

I'm tired today but not feeling sick so I get up and wander round the house doing some bits of cleaning and sitting down at regular times. By early afternoon I need to sleep. I lie on the sofa and start to drift off to be woken by Trevor asking me about the new bathroom lights. I answer him and start to drift off again then another question and another so I give up on sleeping. I do a bit more wandering around then I really do have to sleep but its now gone 3 o'clock and Sally the nurse will be in soon to give me my injection. So I lay on the bed to rest and watch TV to keep me awake.

I jump, Sally jumps in fact I think the whole world jumped as she says hello and taps me gently on the shoulder. So much for not falling asleep, so much for being allowed to go to sleep. Who needs rest anyway I'm only ill you know!

At about 7:00pm I turn over in bed and have a sharp pain in my groin area. I feel and find a small lump under the skin. We decide to phone Exeter hospital and speak to the sister on the cancer ward. She first suggests that I make an appointment with my doctor in the morning then says it might be better if I see a doctor tonight else I probably won't sleep. I know I won't sleep, so off to hospital we go.

We get to the hospital at 8:00pm and of course my notes are in a different hospital and the doctor is covering numerous wards so there will be a wait but it would not be the same if you went to hospital and they saw you straight away would it! I must mention that the welcome onto the ward was warm and relaxed and we were immediately taken to a room with chairs TV and offered coffee.

At 9:10 the doctor arrives and takes me to a bed to examine me. I think nothing now of dropping my trousers and showing whoever my private parts, it's just like showing my arm now. The doctor has a good push around and says she thinks it is an in growing hair follicle. I hope she's right! She tells me that to be on the safe side she will refer me to the Cherry brook day case unit and someone will phone me tomorrow with an appointment for Monday. I feel reassured by what I have been told and head home to bed maybe I can and will be allow to sleep now.

16th October 2006

After a weekend trying not to let my mind wonder and think about the possibility that the cancer has spread because every lump that comes up is automatically cancer now. Monday arrives and the lump has got smaller.

We go off to the hospital, first calling into the Force cancer support building. This is our first visit to this service and we immediately feel relaxed. We are both offered complimentary therapies and both opt for six sessions of aromatherapy.

After a cup of coffee and a wander around their lovely garden it's time to go to my appointment at Cherrybrook to found out what the lump is.

I don't have to wait long before my name is called and I am taken to a bed to await the doctor. I hear my name mentioned several times outside the door then the doctor arrives. He says that the swabs taken on the 12th are not back yet so they will not be doing anything today. He says he will phone me at home if I need some antibiotics. I leave the hospital feeling unsure what might be wrong with me, but decide that if they are not that worried about the lump, then neither should I be.

18th October 2006

Off to Charing Cross today. I am starting to become rebellious in my cancer and we don't leave home until 8:45am instead of 7:15 am! Sadly during the journey I decide to do some research and write down every service station on the route to check them off when we have visited them. So here goes

Exeter services	
Cullompton services	
Tiverton services	
Taunton services	visited
Bridgewater services	
Sedgemoor services	
Gordano services	visited
Leigh delamare services	visited
Membury services	visited
Cheveley services	visited (not going there again, as you can't leave!)
Reading services	
Heston services	visited

I arrive at 1:30pm, book into the ward and quickly leave for the hospital restaurant. I would stay for the ward lunch but I'm not that sick!

My bed is ready on my return to the ward. There is the usual round of doctors and the good news is that my Beta HCG is now 11. They are changing my anti sickness tablets but only have 9 of the anti sickness tablets that work for me in the hospital. I wonder if I should go to the chemist and get some for them, but I'm ill you know!

I feel that I am calmer now I know the routine and it is not long before the chemo is started. This time I feel a lot more tired during the evening and sleep right through the night. They appear to be more organised with my tablets this time and have already put the request into pharmacy for the tablets I need to take home. I think they are lulling me into a false sense of security!

By 11:30am I am ready to go and yes I was right my tablets are not ready.

We leave at 1:00pm and I am as usual asleep before we leave London. I awake at Cullompton with the rain pouring down and request a toilet stop (another service station completed!).

Home again and I fall into bed and it is not long before I'm asleep again. Part of the tablet change involves taking one pill every six hours for four days. So I set the alarm which reminds minds me of having small children, wasn't that where this all started?

20th October 2006

I don't feel too bad today. The new anti sickness tablets seem to be working and I'm not too tired. Trevor has decided to start the bathroom tiling today and I am determined to help. I am the chief tile cutter. After an hour I am knackered so sit down between tile cuttings but do not give in to the tiredness. I manage to eat a sandwich but the mouthwash after makes me sick. I know that I have to carry on with the mouthwash or else the ulcers and thrush could return and what's a little sick between friends!

Bed can't come soon enough and I'm asleep by 9:00pm, awake by 12:00 for a tablet, then awake by 6:00am for another tablet. So much for resting! Could they not make time release tablets so you don't have to get up in the night?

22nd October 2006

I'm feeling fed up today. I just want some time without cancer. It feels like it is ruling my life and I don't want it to. Just a small amount of time would be enough to get rid of this feeling but I know that this is not possible at present.

The bathroom tiling is going well and takes my mind off the cancer for a while. However I am well aware how tired I get in a short space of time. After completing one wall of tiles (mainly sat watching Trevor work) yesterday I was in bed by 7:00pm and asleep by 7:30pm, and then awake at 12 and 6am for tablets.

The district nurse yesterday asked if I wanted to learn how to give my own injections, is she mad! Why would I want to inflict pain on myself? I think that by the time I had plucked up courage to get the needle close to my arm I would pass out. I'm not good with needles but with the amount of blood tests I am having I will soon be able to drink a glass of water and become a fountain!

24th October 2006

I feel as though I have more energy today and I am sure going to use it. So I spend the day racing around doing everything that most people would do in a week. I feel I need to do this because I know the next few days I will not want to do anything.

I visit my nephews who have not seen me without hair yet. My 5 year old nephew looks at me and my blue hat and asks if I have blue hair now! They have been told that I have my other hair (Nina). I tell them that my hair is like their cousins hair who is a few weeks old. Next minute the conversation is about something completely different and the subject is closed.

25th October 2006

I have an appointment to meet the consultant in Exeter today but of course it is not the only medical appointment. Added to this I am still very tired from the last chemo and yes it is chemo day again. At 8:30 I have my sinus hole dressed by Melissa at the doctors. Then off to hospital to see the consultant at 9:30 and to finish the morning, chemo. Life is such a whirlwind!

After meeting my Exeter consultant I'm off to Cherrybrook for chemo where the nurse who gave me my chemo a fortnight ago asks me if I have been behaving. I replied 'if you can't misbehave when you have cancer when can you?' she laughs and agrees so I now have the medical approval to misbehave!

I arrive home at 1:00pm and by 1:30 I am asleep. I awake at 6:00pm feeling sick and still tired. I decide to try and eat some tea, which tastes nice until about five minutes after I have finished it then I regret eating anything.

I spend the rest of the evening trying not to think about feeling sick but the more I try the worse I feel. By 10:00 I'm asleep again having not needed the sick bowl. I am spending more and more time asleep each day. I know that the effects of the chemo are accumulative but I wish they weren't as I have a life to live.

26th October 2006

I wake at 8:00am still feeling sick and still tired. I'm not even going to try to get out of bed today. I lay in bed feeling sorry for myself and why shouldn't I, I'm ill you know.

I decide to entertain myself by filling another form from the department of Work and Pensions. Can life get any better? You need to have time off being sick to fill in all the forms!

Then Becky arrives with a present for me. It's my wig for my brother's party, a long sparkly wig, and well if you've got no hair why not!

I put the wig on at the same time Sally the nurse arrives to give me my injection. She takes one look at me and says she won't be able to take me seriously again. I ask 'did you before?' 'No' she replies. I decide that they have allocated me the right nurse to see me through my cancer.

I manage to eat some tea which at present is staying down. Let's hope it stays there tonight.

p.s. my beta HCG is now 10.

27ᵗʰ *October 2006*

This is the first day that I feel like phoning the doctors surgery and telling Melissa I am not well enough to attend my appointment. I struggle out of bed and make my way to the doctors still feeling sick. I now know what fatigue is. I ache all over and just putting one foot in front of another is an effort. Being the independent person that I am, I turn down Trevor's offer to drive me to the surgery, which is a mistake. I hold my arm out for Melissa to take the blood test and tell her I want to crawl up in a ball under a duvet and be left alone. I lay down for the sinus dressing to be done and wish I was somewhere else. After returning to my car I turn around to meet Melissa carrying the dressing pack that I left in the surgery. Maybe I was somewhere else.

I return home shattered. I sit on the settee for much of the rest of the morning occasionally getting up to do some housework but by early afternoon I have to lie down in bed.

I am awoken by Sally the nurse to have my injection. She has tried to talk Trevor into waking me up after the last episode of nearly giving herself and me a heart attack, but he also has a sense of humour and leaves her to it! I tell her how I felt this morning and she says that I can always ring her if I don't feel like going out. Why didn't I think of that? I still can't get my head around how ill I am. I just carry on with life and forget that I have a serious illness instead of using the help that is there for me.

The hot flushes have returned which feels strange when you have a bald head. The heat rises through my body and then explodes out of my head which feels hot and then cold at the same time, work that one out. I am not able to have HRT treatment because the type of cancer I have feeds on oestrogen. Well what did I expect that life would be easy?

Something very serious has just happened. After tea I ask for some chocolate ice cream. It tastes of metal. The world is definitely not at one if chocolate does not taste right. Should I be admitted into hospital by air ambulance? I know that I was told that my taste buds would change but they did not tell me what a devastating effect this could have on my life!

It's strange that although I feel sick, I am still hungry. In fact when I eat and for a while after the sickness goes. How does that work?

28ᵗʰ *October 2006*

I spend most of the day resting as tonight is my Brother Simon's 40ᵗʰ birthday party and I am going come what may.

We arrive at 8:00pm with me in a sparkly wig (well if you have no hair it must be done!) to be met by my eight year old nephew George and his five year old brother Harry who announces that I am wearing my other hair.

My family have all put together and paid for Simon to be driven at high speed around a race track in a Ferrari. I had wrapped it up in a large incontinence pad just in case he needs to wear one!

I get lots of support from friends who are there and manage one dance then I'm knackered. I decide to volunteer as the photographer for the night.

I have had a great evening and survive until 11:45pm then give into the tiredness and go home. I fall into bed and know I will pay for this for the next few days but I would not have missed it for the world.

29ᵗʰ October 2006

Yes I'm paying for the night before. Getting out of bed is a problem. I tried it once, didn't like it, and so went back to bed. My muscles ache all over and I haven't even run a marathon. But then my muscles ache most days. I also feel sick most days, that kind of feeling where you know you won't be sick you just feel sick.

I spend most of the day in bed and sleep for two hours in the afternoon which is becoming the norm now.

4:00pm and Sally arrives to change my dressing and give me my injection.

At night I take pain killers to relieve the muscle ache. The tablets dull the pain but don't take the whole pain away, but I'm too exhausted not to sleep.

30ᵗʰ October 2006

I wake feeling sorry for myself. I am beginning to realise that I am not recovering between chemo's and not getting the two good days before the next treatment.

My muscles still hurt and getting out of bed is just too much for me. I know that I need to do something to get myself through the day as hiding under the duvet is not a good place to be.

I decide to phone the doctors and ask for an appointment to talk to Gilly. Gilly had said right at the beginning of my diagnosis if I need to talk then ring her, so I'm taking her at her word.

I get an appointment at 3:00pm, so stay in bed till then of course having my usual sleep before I go. I sit and tell her that I am exhausted and I just want a week's holiday where no one stabs or prods me. We both know this is not possible at the moment.

I am reassured to hear her say that I am going through a really tough chemo regime as they are going for a cure and she is not surprised I am exhausted. I know how tough this is as I am the one who is living it but the acknowledgement and empathy of the situation calms me.

She says that I should do one nice thing for myself each day however small it is and to hold onto the holiday I can have when the chemo has ended.

I can feel the tears behind my eyes but they don't flow.

The hug at the end is very welcome in fact I could do with more of them.

I return home feeling a bit lighter after talking to Gilly and know I can call on her again if needed.

The thought of having more chemo in London is beyond me at the moment and I know I should be talking to Linda about how I feel but that is just one conversation too far. In fact just thinking about the chemo makes me taste the chemicals in my mouth.

I appear to have lost my sense of humour at present. This shows me that I am not good at the moment. I'm sure it will return given time but until then I'm off to my bed to feel sorry for myself and I have every right too!

31st October 2006

Well so much for telling Gilly how well I am sleeping! It's now 5:43 am and I'm wide awake but the good news is the sense of humour has returned. I woke up wandering if there was a total eclipse of the moon then realised that my eyelids were stuck together! As I have now lost most of my eye lashes the dirt sticks to my eyelids and regularly has the above effect. As Trevor says 'it's all part of it!'

I have again decamped to the front room and get to watch the early morning telly. There is a grown man showing me how to build a level crossing on a H.O scale model railway. It is apparently important to make sure that the gate posts are drilled in straight or the gates won't open you know. 'Get a life' springs to mind but I can see the amount of enjoyment on his little smiling face so I decide to leave him alone in his own world.

As for me, life feels a bit brighter than yesterday. I don't feel so sick and my muscles don't ache too much at the moment. I haven't told Trevor yet (I don't think he would like to be woken up yet!) but the nice thing for me today is to go and have a cup of tea at the beach, maybe even a small walk on the sand if I'm good! I know that I am not able to drive the 10 miles to the beach so I hope Trevor is able to leave the bathroom tiling to take me. I'm sure he will tear himself away!

Well I made it to the beach and we also had lunch with a friend in a pub which was great.

However back at home I crawl back into bed exhausted from the morning's exhaustions. I sleep until 4:00pm

I phone for my blood results which are fine. So definitely off to Charing Cross hospital tomorrow for some more poison. Although I know I need the chemo in the back off my mind a week off would be good, but if that happened I would be wanting the Chemo so I can't win.

I have realised that I have not informed you of our understanding of the medical terms used by the doctors. There have been so many that we have resorted to our own language. You will find our glossary at the back of this book (because that's where they always are!).

In the evening Becky suggests that I am used to frighten the children away during trick or treat. I am to be the trick. She wants to dress me up but leave my head bald, and place me outside the front door as she is sure this would be scarier than anything they could do! Children these days!

1st November 2006

Charing Cross here we come again. This time we leave at 9:00am it's getting later each time and do you know what I don't care!

Just outside Maidenhead we get caught in a traffic jam and the guilt almost sets in that we should have left earlier. I ask Jane Satnav for an alternative route but by the time she sorts herself out we are past the accident and on our way again. I ask Trevor if he wants Tim Satnav back but the look is enough for me to leave Jane on.

There are no permit parking spaces in the hospital so we have to park outside. If you knew Trevor's sense of direction you would be as worried as I am about him moving the car later!

Yes the bed is not ready, but it won't be long I'm told. Trevor goes for lunch, I already feel sick due to he smell of the chemo on the ward so sit in the day room. They were right; my bed was not long before it was ready. Trevor goes off to move the car I hope to see him later today!

The doctor arrives and tells me the good news that my Beta HCG level in now 4 and normal. I ask if he will put in writing that I am normal which he declines and says he is willing to write that my blood is normal. You just can't get the doctors these days!

He also says that they will give me another 8 chemo's just to make sure the cancer has gone. Well aren't I the lucky one!

2nd *November 2006*

My chemo is finished by 11:00am and behold, my tablets are here by 12:00, see miracles do happen! So off we go back home.

Jane Satnav is having a bad day, maybe she is premenstrual! She tries to send us the wrong way off the roundabout but we are not that stupid and go the right way! This time I don't even mention Tim Satnav as Trevor is already stressed by Jane.

We stop at Reading services which is another off the list. I buy some pineapple which is wonderful and sweet and I thoroughly enjoy eating it. I am asleep within minutes of leaving the services. I awake a few miles from our house and ask 'are we nearly there yet?'

I fall into bed feeling very sick. By 6:10pm I am being sick. It's lucky I ate the pineapple or what would I have brought up! I know that I will not be able to keep my 7:00pm tablet down and without this tablet the thrush and mouth ulcers will return, so I ask Trevor to phone the doctor to get an anti-sickness injection.

The doctor arrives and stabs me in the bum, so now I have a sore bum as well. I take my tablet and I am soon asleep. I awake with a start and wonder why the alarm has not gone off at 1:00am for the next tablet. This will be because it is only 10:45pm. I'm sure that injection had hallucinatory powers!

3rd November 2006

The alarm does go off at 1:00am and then 7:00am. I spend most off the day in bed, sleeping on and off. The nurse arrives at 4:00pm to give me my GCSF Injection.

We are due to go to what has become an annual firework display with friends. It involves eating sausages and watching three grown men making firework lighting a true art (mainly abstract art!). I am determined not to miss this spectacular so drag myself out of bed. I am so glad I made the effort as the laughter did not stop. At one point everyone was trying to disguise themselves by pulling hats over there heads I decided that my better option was to take my hat off as who would recognise a bald women?

We return home at 9:45pm and I am exhausted but in much better spirits and I don't feel sick which has to be a bonus.

I would also like it to be known that I consumed no alcohol! In fact I have had no alcohol for months now.

I should also mention here (much to my children's disgust I suspect) that the sex life is not well. I asked Sally a week ago if it was possible to resume marital relations. Well what I did ask her was to make no remarks just a "yes" or "no" would do. With a smile on her face she said yes. I asked her to leave the room as it has been three months but she continued on with the dressing! It's not that I don't fancy Trevor anymore I'm just so knackered most of the time. My mind is willing but my body is not! So much for 'you can have sex during treatment!'

When we do resume marital relationship I do find it difficult to relax after all the medical experiences I have had and the fear that my body may not be up to it. If I ever feel like sex again maybe the fears will be gone.

4th *November 2006*

Today has been a very frustrating one. I want to do so much but just the thought of getting out of bed is too much. I want to help with the floor tiles and do some housework. I just want to get Trevor some lunch as he is working so hard. I walk to the kitchen open the fridge door and shut it again knowing that I cannot cope with even making a sandwich. So I fall back into bed and Trevor gets my lunch for me. I spend the rest of the day in bed, feeling sorry for myself.

The department of work and pensions has sent me a letter saying that they have still not decided if I qualify for disability living allowance. This also means that Trevor cannot claim carer's allowance. They have had a letter from my doctor and a letter from my surgeon both with my cancer diagnosis. How ill do you have to be to get it? If I was dead do you think I might qualify then! If they think that Trevor is not caring for me then they should spend a day with me and see just how little I can do.

By the time the district nurse arrives I have convinced myself that the sinus hole is getting bigger. I ask her as she redresses it. She says its not but I'm not sure she is right which is silly as I can't see the hole and she can!

It is very difficult not to let the frustration get to me so in the evening I get myself out of bed to sit on the sofa and watch TV. I am unable to sit still and feel very unsettled, about what I don't know. The more I try to relax the worse I get so off back to bed I go. I take some pain killers for the muscle aches and eventually relax enough to sleep.

5th November 2006

Today I feel that I have more energy. And when I say I am having a good day to anyone else this would be a bad day for example I manage to complete 10 minutes of housework and then sit down for ½ an half to rest!

It is firework night and after the suggestions about Halloween I am staying in for fear of being put on the bonfire as the Guy!

The frustration is getting worse and I am unable to sleep until 3:40am. I keep going over in my head what I want to do tomorrow but I know that it is less likely that I will manage anything if I don't go to sleep.

6th November 2006

I am a little tired today (yes this is an understatement!). The morning is taken up by medical appointments and shopping of course this is with the aid of Trevor. One day when I have grown up I will be able to go out by myself!

I ask Melissa if she thinks the sinus hole is bigger. She says it is longer not deeper. So I'm not going mad (no comments here!). Melissa suggests I use needle and cotton to sew it up but that would hurt I reply 'I'll use superglue'.

I am unwilling to give in to the tiredness so push myself throughout the day. I now know that the days I feel like I can do things I push myself to hard, but I also know that for about four days after Wednesday's chemo I will not be up to much.

It's a day without any medical interventions tomorrow. This is very rare and I'm going to make the most of it. The only problem at the moment is that I have a runny nose. I will keep an eye on my temperature and hope that I don't have to go back to A &E to be told I have a cold again.

I am still working when it's bedtime. Trevor suggests that I take a couple of pain killers before I go to bed. My muscles ache so much of the time now that I don't take much notice of them however after last nights lack of sleep I will try anything.

I'll let you know in the morning if the tablets work

7ᵗʰ *November 2006*

No the tablets didn't work! I did sleep until 4:23am but the pain from my muscles awoke me. I can't take any other tablets until I have checked out with Linda at Charing Cross whether they are safe for me to take while on Chemo. Unfortunately that will not be until about 9:30am so I make a cup of tea for Trevor and myself. Of course it is educational TV time. This morning I am blessed with the knowledge of how to massage a beluga to release the caviar without having to kill the fish; I'll test my technique out on our goldfish later!

At 10:00am I bleep Linda and she suggests a different kind of painkiller which I already had in the house. In fact at present I think I probably have more supplies in the house than the Chemist. The muscle pain is to do with the GCSF injections, Linda tells me. Well that's a relief.

Linda has been reading a copy of this book up to 25th October she says that this book is a revelation as I am sharing a lot more writing than I say. My doctor at Charing Cross has also read it and has recognised himself in it. So maybe I should tell you his name if I could only remember how to say it. I will ask how he pronounces and spells his name when I see him next and include him in dispatches.

Colleen comes to see me today as I am not able to get myself going enough to visit her. As usual the laughter rings through the house and Trevor tells her he is now calling me 'his little slap head' what terms of endearment he has. I would be rude back to him but I want the bathroom finished! You see although I may not be physically able, my mouth is still working.

On the bathroom front it's looking smashing. Unfortunately the basin looks the same as it has smashed in half and is all over the floor! I am not bothered about details like this anymore in fact I think it's funny! A while ago something like the basin smashing or Trevor being involved in the situation would have left me running around like a headless chicken and blaming everyone. Now it's not important. Living is important and taking one day at a time is how I am coping with life at the moment.

I'm going to take one of the strong painkillers now before bed. I'll let you know in the morning if the tablets work!

8ᵗʰ *November 2006*

Well it's getting better this morning I have slept until 5:40am. My muscles don't hurt as much today but don't get too excited as its chemo day so the cycle starts again.

Did you know that they had to build a shed the size of 75 football pitches to construct the Boeing 747! Yes it's early morning TV again.

I am refilled with dressing and then it's off for chemo in Exeter. My chemo nurse, Lizzie wishes to be mentioned in this book and assures me that she will be at the book signing. She tells me to write that she is thin and good looking (the pigs are flying!) she seems to think that I could be trouble. I don't know how she got that idea!

I am tired again now after all the chemicals and know that tomorrow I will not move far from home. I have a phone call from the Force Cancer centre who offer Trevor and myself a aromatherapy massage at 1:00pm tomorrow and although I think I might struggle to get there it will do the aching muscles good. Trevor still seems sceptical about the aromatherapy. I don't know what he thinks they are going to do to him but I am sure that afterwards it will be the best thing he has ever had! I'll let you know how he gets on.

I have decided to hire myself out for quiz nights as with all the knowledge I am gaining from early morning TV I would be an asset to any team. Knowledge is power so they say, well with all this power you would think I would be able to sleep!

9ᵀᴴ *November 2006*

I have spent most of the day in bed. My only outing was for the aromatherapy. Yes Trevor really enjoyed his and it was not what he was expecting! In fact he is even thinking about attending the relaxation classes.

I also enjoyed mine it helped for a short time to relieve the aching muscles but I am soon to resort back to the pills.

I feel sick all day and really look forward to my injection which will add to the flu symptoms!

I am now receiving 'hand me ups' from my children as all of my clothes are miles too big for me. I have lost lots of weight and the 'c' plan diet (cancer plan) is working. Well I needed to lose a few stone!

My wedding ring does not fit either. If I wash my hands my ring falls off, so I have decided not to wear it in case I lose it. The wonderful Trevor has brought me another ring and spent all of £3:50 on me! I will have my wedding ring resized when all this is over.

When the nurse arrives to give me the injection I really want to tell her I don't want it today but I know that without it my chemo could be postponed and as I am doing so well that would be stupid so the injection it is.

I must admit I am doing a very good 'poor me' today if only for my own benefit. Well if I can't do it now when can I?

10ᵗʰ November 2006

And I still feel sick! But I get myself out of bed, go and have the hole dressed, and of course a blood test.

On my return home I am exhausted but refuse to let myself lie in bed again, well that was a good thought until 12:00ish when the pull to bed became to much and sleep beckons. After 2 ½ hours I am awake again and guess what still feeling sick! Trying to take my mind off the nausea and aching I decide to try to link the computer to the internet. After 2 hours I have decided that rather than have a headache from banging my head against the wall I'll put up with feeling sick!

When the nurse arrives at 4:00pm to give me my injection I tell her that I could do without it today. So I have it anyway!

I think that my body thermostat has malfunctioned! I am cold most of the time. I don't think that we are aware how much insulation our body hair gives us. Well I am now! Last night I went to bed with the central heating on and a hot water bottle. The coldness goes right into my bones and getting warmed up takes a long time. Can you get a whole body wig?

Another problem that I have developed is that I forget words. This is not something I had a problem with before the cancer. It is not necessarily difficult words in fact it is quite often words that I use all the time for example I was talking to someone earlier and forgot the word magazine. I have decided to put this problem down to the fatigue.

11ᵗʰ November 2006

I must have grown up today as I am going out by myself. Well when I say out within 2 miles of my home but I am driving myself. I spend time with my friend Pat, at her house helping with the village pantomime. I am gutted that I am unable to take part this year and I am missing the rehearsal nights. I would love to have been on stage again this year but at least I can help in some ways. I have asked if there are any parts for an overgrown baby with a bald head, but apparently Aladdin does not have this role! Maybe next year.

In the afternoon I try to do some gardening. I manage to wrap 3 plants in fleece for the winter and that is it. As I have said before my mouth still works and the rest of the gardening is done by Trevor under my supervision!

Back to the house and I am exhausted. That's me finished for the day. Well apart from the afternoon injection.

I forgot to mention that I am now trained in ship building. If you ever want the Queen Mary 2 built call me (more early morning TV). For those of you who are not watching TV at the same times as me you don't know what you are missing, Or maybe you do!

Apart from now feeling exhausted I do not feel sick today. That means I have 4 days before I feel sick again. Who said I didn't have anything to look forward too.

It's now early evening and I already know that I will need pain killers again to soothe the muscle aches before I go to bed. This also means that I will need to take something to help with my bowels. I think that I take as many tablets to counteract the effects of the chemo as the chemo chemicals themselves.

12ᵗʰ November 2006

The muscle pain wakes me again and I decide that I am not decamping to the front room again. So I take more tablets and Trevor makes me a cup of tea. I lie in bed and try to relax but all I am doing is thinking what I will write in this damn book. So I give in and go to the front room and open up the computer.

But really I am not angry with the book I am angry and frustrated by not being able to do much. Yes I am slightly angry with life! All I want is my energy back. I want a holiday. I want to be able do some gardening without being tired after 5 minutes. I don't want to feel sick most of the time. I don't want my muscles to ache. I don't want any more injections and yes I am ranting but I'm ill you know!

I drop off back to sleep until the Archers which is a tradition for Sunday mornings in this house. My youngest daughter, Vicky and her partner Richard are coming to lunch. Normally I would have been able to cook the lunch by myself but this is not possible due to the fatigue. So Trevor helps. After lunch I don't have any choice but to go to bed and sleep. I awake when the nurse arrives for my afternoon injection. Vicky and Richard have left. I wasn't even able to be awake long enough to say goodbye. This makes me sad as I am beginning to see how much effect the chemo is having on my life.

Although I don't feel sick there is a funny taste in my mouth. This is there most of the time now and I can't describe what it is like. The only word that comes to mind is stale. Maybe I'm going off!

13ᵗʰ *November 2006*

Another painful awaking and some more early morning TV. This morning I have learnt that you can strip wallpaper with fabric softener, so goodness knows what it does to your clothes!

I am supposed to be going out with Caroline, my sister-in-law today, but know this is not possible as just getting out of bed for the toilet is enough. So Trevor rings to cancel this and I spend the morning in bed. I am fed up as I was really looking forward to the day out after our last shopping expedition. Caroline had chosen another town for us to visit. I suspect that we were probably banned from the last one due to all the laughter!

I talk to Linda on the phone as the hospital accommodation is fully booked. Trevor does not seem too keen on sleeping in the car so I ask for some alternative bed and breakfasts names. I also mention about my memory problems. She assures me that this is due to the chemo. So it's not Alzheimer's then!

My fatigue could get worse she tells me. Well that's another thing to look forward too. Does this mean I will sleep mornings and afternoons? That will be alright as long as it does not affect my early morning learning!

I said that I would mention in dispatches the name of my doctor in Charing Cross well it's Myooran. I am expecting him to put the cheque in the post for this mention soon!

In the afternoon our car needs fixing and I don't feel that I can stay home alone or cope with being out at a garage for 2 hours. So I phone a friend and arrange to go there for the afternoon. I sit down in her lounge and that's where I stay until Trevor arrives to take me home again. Even this is exhausting. It's now 7:43pm and I am already thinking about going to bed. This had better all be worth going through or someone is going to be in big trouble!

17ᵗʰ *November 2006*

Yes I know I haven't written anything for a few days but I'm ill you know! Well really I felt like I was beginning to rant and that is not what this book is about. However on reflection I now realise that I felt like life was going round in circles. The same old thing was happening every day. This involved me mainly sleeping, getting frustrated with myself and going to medical appointments. That's what cancer is like it takes over your life. It's up to me to take control back and yes I know that it is all I seem to live and breathe at the moment but there are ways that I can have breaks from the cancer, for example writing this book, doing what I can around the house when I feel like it and doing something nice for me each day (see I do listen to others!).

I have had another dose of chemo at Charing Cross on the 15th. I had to push myself to go this time but this time the after effects have not been too bad. Myooran has changed my anti-sickness medication and it seems to be working. My Beta HCG is 6 which is fine as apparently it does 'bob' up and down a bit (obviously bob is a medical term!). I am also given 2 units of blood as my blood count has dropped and I am anaemic. This accounts for some of the fatigue. According to Linda I am 'a whiter shade of pale!'

Only one slight problem is the wound is getting bigger and very smelly so I now need it dressed daily for a while. Trevor asks Myooran if this is typical of a hysterectomy scar. Myooran replies that I am not a typical patient. I will take this remark as the compliment it was obviously meant to be!

I was wondering what I could do with my one day off of medical interventions a week and now the problem is solved, I have a dressing done!

I would like to thank the staff of Charing cross for providing the light entertainment during my stay and returning my sense of humour again.

Scene 1

Linda and Myooran enter a small room called the Intrathecal room off the ward I was on with a patient. There then followed a in and out the door scene. Linda places what looked like 2 pink Barbie lunch boxes outside the door. She then opens that door again to retrieve the chemo syringe that she needed. Myooran leaves the room to wash his hands then can't get back in the room as he can't touch the door handle with his clean hands. The patient is then pushed out of the room on her bed. Linda had forgotten to draw herself one of her legendary maps and crashes the bed into a trolley.

Scene 2

Linda comes to ask me how I am. Trevor had put some laces on the table as his laces were too long and he needed to replace them. He was unable to cut them having no scissors so on the table they stayed. Linda said she had to ask why there were shoe laces on the table. I replied that I thought you needed to remove your shoe laces in case of suicidal thoughts. Trevor explained the real reason and then Linda said to Trevor 'shall I give you one?' although Trevor and Linda tried to ignore this remark I am not that discreet and laugh. Linda taps me on the foot and tells me I am wicked!

Well I wasn't the one who offered to give him one!

Scene 3

A doctor enters my room and presses the hand wash dispenser down. Unfortunately instead of the liquid flowing slowly into his hands it shoots out at a 90 degree angle and covered his shirt from top to bottom. He reacted by saying he was not impressed by the dispenser. I said I was very impressed and laughed. He said he was happy to entertain the patients and left to clean his shirt.

Scene 4

A repeat of the above by Myooran. After examining my wound and needed to wash his hands. I nearly managed to tell him about the dispenser but I blame my lack of warning on my short term memory loss!

I would also like to update you with the latest service station count!

Exeter services	
Cullompton services	visited
Tiverton services	
Taunton services	visited
Bridgewater services	
Sedgemoor services	visited

Gordano services	visited
Leigh delamare services	visited
Membury	visited
Cheveley services	visited (not going there again, as you can't leave!)
Reading services	visited
Heston services	visited

Only 3 service stations to go. Exeter could be a problem as we only live 4 miles from it. Trevor says we can visit it on our last London chemo, just for the hell of it!

After yesterdays blood I do feel like I have more energy. By this I mean that I don't need to sleep during the day. Getting out of bed for any length of time is still too much.

Sally is back from her holiday and arrives to give me my injection and dress the wound. The wound is clean today and not smelly so I am very pleased that I am not going rotten.

When I said Sally was back from her holiday I must have meant in body as she has left her bag behind, I will put a sign on it to tell people where to return the bag when she does it again as I am a helpful person sometimes and I know she will thank me for the help given time. I thought I was the one with the short term memory loss!

Speaking of my short term memory I have just realised that I am still wearing my hospital armband. Maybe I should keep it on to remind me of my name in case of an emergency!

18th November 2006

I have slept for 12 hours so no early morning TV, but that does not mean that my education has stopped. Trevor has invented a new use for hospital sick bowls. He is mixing the tile grout in one! Could the NHS make money by selling this product to the building trade at marked up prices?

I have remained in bed for the morning and feel a lot more relaxed about resting. Maybe all the ranting has got some of the frustration out of my system. I get up in the afternoon and walk down to our pond at the bottom of the garden with hot drinks for Trevor and I. By the time I get there it is raining so I go back up the steps to the house. I am now exhausted and breathing heavily. Well that's today's exercise over.

The nurse arrives, she recognises me. It turns out our daughters went to the same school together. She gives me my injection and changes my dressing. I also am bleeding under the skin on the back of my left hand. This is where the cannula was put in the wrong place at Charing Cross on Wednesday.

The nurse phones the duty doctor for advice and then draws in black pen around the red area so I can see if it spreads. I now have a mark like the scarlet pimpernel or maybe it's the Black Death, bring out your dead!

I should also point out that this book that I was not going to write is just over 21,000 words! How did that happen? I still blame my doctor! Just don't tell him I am enjoying writing this.

19th November 2006

I am going out today even if it kills me. I want to do some Christmas shopping. I did most of it last night on the internet. Family and friends will just have to have what I can buy easily this year as I know that walking around Exeter with the world and his wife will be too much for me.

Trevor and I drive to a local shop but we are unable to park the car in their car park. This then involves a walk to the shop of about 100 metres (50 yards in English money!). I walk once around the shop then back to the car and I am exhausted. So we return home.

I'm starting to feel a bit depressed not sure why. I just am. All I want to do is have a relaxing bath but with the wound still open it is not a good idea.

By 7:00pm I am ready for bed. The other routine I have not told you about is my hot water bottle. My feet seem to get very cold when I go to bed. In fact I would call them icy cold which goes right into my bones. They take about an hour to warm up again and if I keep the hot water bottle any longer than that the hot flushes feel worse. I would be hot stuff if I had any form of sex drive left!

20ᵗʰ *November 2006*

Well where shall I start. I manage the morning well. We meet my dad and step mum for coffee and ordered the new carpet for the front room. Of course there was the trip to Melissa for bloods to be taken and a dressing done.

The afternoon has been a different matter. I feel like I could cry but I am not sure that I want to. I don't even know what I would be crying about. I just feel low. I ask Trevor not to tell Sally when she comes to give my injection, so he does.

When she asks me how I am I tell her the truth that I feel like I have had enough and one more chemo is one too many. Sally talks to me about the end is now in sight and maybe my body is ready to let go as up till now the adrenaline has kept me going. Now that adrenaline is not needed so much and I am able to think about what I have been going through.

I explain to her how when others tell me how hard the chemo regime that I am on is, it does not feel that tough to me as I am just getting on with it. It's just how life is for me.

Now that I am not able to do very much each day I do have more time to think and yes I do think that Sally is right in a way. I am now allowing myself to sit with all the feelings that I have not made time for in the past few months. I know I am not out of the woods yet but it does feel like a safer place to be at the moment as there was I time when I did not think I would make it to Christmas.

I am still scared that this might all go wrong. I am also overwhelmed by sadness for myself because of all I have been through over the past few months. The pain both physical and emotional; the uncertainty of what will happen; the being strong for others; the pulling myself through each day when I would rather have just curled up under the duvet; the exhaustion, the fatigue and the frustration.

I also feel that I should really be celebrating the fact that my Beta HCG is now back to normal and my prognosis is good, but I can't yet.

I ring Linda to check the results of the swab that was taken last week from my wound. Linda tells me that I have an infection and Myooran says I need antibiotics. I ask Linda to thank Myooran, which she does. Linda arranges with Kieran for me to pick up a prescription tomorrow and the antibiotics may make me feel sick. I thank Linda for that and say goodbye. What I really wanted to say to her is I am struggling here, but I don't and regret it afterwards.

So now I'm off to my bed with my hot water bottle and it's my party and I can cry if I want to.

21st November 2006

So it wasn't my party and I didn't cry even though I wanted to!

I heard from a friend, Pat today that one of the pantomime cast has had to pull out and my mind immediately went into over drive. I desperately want to be a part of the cast and convince myself that I will be alright by the beginning of February to take part. I am even planning to phone the producer and offer my services.

It takes Trevor to sit down and tell me that I will not be well enough or have the amount of energy to go on stage for six performances. I don't want to hear this but I know that he is right.

Another day over and I am so looking forward to another chemo session tomorrow (not).

22nd November 2006

My first stop is the surgery to be repacked by Melissa who is now a year older and vast amounts of money will stop me mentioning her age! I make my appointments for next week and comment to the receptionist that my social diary would be empty without cancer. She seems a bit shocked that I have said that, I can't think why!

Chemo is at 11:45 and Lizzie again wishes to be mentioned as she says that one mention is good but two mentions will show that we have a 'good rapport!' I tell her that I will tell the truth about her bodily stature but this is difficult to do when she is just about to stab you in the hand with a cannula.

I ask to speak to her in a separate room. I tell her that I have a bit of night incontinence. She contacts the doctor who says that it could be to do with my body readjusting to the new shape internally and to not drink too much caffeine or alcohol at night. This could be a problem as I am not drinking alcohol at all. Maybe I should start!

The chemo goes ahead and I am soon home and back in bed.

I haven't as yet mentioned the cost of cancer. Although health care in this country is free I have had to fight to get my trips to London paid for, plus Trevor's accommodation costs while I am in London. At present we have paid out just over £600 and that does not include the new wardrobe I will need to buy due to my 'c' plan diet!

The bathroom is finished. Just thought you ought to know and yes it looks stunning.

I apologise but my memory is not good so here is an update. You can clean a rusty bath with coco-cola (yes it works as we have tried it on our bath) thank goodness for early morning TV.

I have made a note to only drink coke when I have the metal taste in my mouth!

Also I think I know why I had the bleeds back in august. The day before the bleeds I booked 2 tickets to see the 'vagina monologues' at the theatre. Should I contact Injury lawyers 4 u and sue the theatre? I'll see if I enjoy it first!

I feel I should share with you the text message I have just received from Jane who has just read these writings, it reads; I have contacted Andrew Lloyd Webber about the musical, it could be called 'Nikki and the scarves of many colours'. Apparently she wants a share in the royalties.

25th November 2006

I'm going to have to change the title of this book as the department of work and pensions has refused my claim for disability living allowance. Apparently I'm not ill enough! So I am going to start taking cocaine, have an alcoholic drink before noon and cut my leg off and then I might be eligible. By the way I might rename the book 'I'm not ill enough you know!' seriously the last thing I want to be doing at present is writing an appeal letter. This is difficult when you have the concentration of o gnat and energy levels of a sloth.

Today I don't feel right, but ask me what is wrong and I can't tell you. I have the usual aches, pains and fatigue, but it's more than that.

I did not sleep well as my mind was in overdrive. I am often feeling very scared that it is all going to go wrong. Once this thought starts going around it is difficult to stop.

I have tried to sleep this afternoon but it was not to be, so tired I stay and look forward to another sleepless night.

26ᵗʰ November 2006

I have spent most of the day composing a letter to the department of work and pensions. I am finding reading it quite hard as it clearly states what my life is like at present.

I have decided to copy the letter into this book, so here goes.

Dear Sir/Madam

I would like to ask you to reconsider your decision about the non award of my disability living allowance for the following reasons.

The original application was submitted on 10/9/2006, since then my medical condition and my ability to cope have deteriorated. I have contacted your department by telephone to update you of my condition, but I am unsure as to whether this information was passed on.

I had a haemorrhage on the 9/8/2006 and was admitted to Exeter hospital I had a further haemorrhage on 10/8/2006 and was again admitted to Exeter hospital.

I had a hysterectomy on 16/8/2006.

I was diagnosed with suspected choriocarcinoma on 16/8/2006 at Exeter and referred to Charing Cross hospital, London due to the rare form of this cancer.

I was admitted to Charing Cross hospital on 11/9/2006 where the diagnosis was confirmed to be choriocarcinoma.

I started chemotherapy treatment on 13/9/2006

My chemotherapy regime is as follows; one week in London for two days where

I receive a fourteen hour chemotherapy (EMA regime) which involves a 344 mile round trip for which my husband drives me, next week Exeter for one day (CO regime). I have to date received ten sessions in eleven weeks (one week off due to infection).

I have severe fatigue due to the effects of the chemotherapy. This stops me from walking anymore than 100 meters without being out of breath. My walking speed has also slowed.

I am not driving my car or using public transport due to dizziness, blurred vision, fatigue and lack of concentration which are all side effects of my chemotherapy regime.

I have recently had bouts of incontinence at night and at present I am experiencing the same difficulties during the day.

I have lost my hair

I am unable to prepare meals for myself for approx four days after my chemotherapy due to the fatigue and lack of concentration.

I am unable to shower or bath at present due to a sinus wound which has opened at the bottom of my hysterectomy scar. This is not healing and I am told is unlikely to heal until after the chemotherapy has finished, due to my low immune system.

The following four days after my chemotherapy treatment I have an injection administered by the district nurse service to boost my white blood cell count, as my blood count does not have time to recover due to the chemotherapy treatment being giving weekly. These injections cause me to suffer from flu like symptoms which include aching muscles for which I take strong painkillers.

I am experiences problems with my short term memory an example of this is having to stop during a conversation because I can't remember words.

After my Charing Cross chemotherapy session I am required to take a course of tablets strictly every six hours for four days. I regularly need reminding to take the tablets due to my short term memory problems.

I have a daily dressing on the sinus wound either at my doctor's surgery (which requires someone to drive me there) or by a district nurse.

I have blood tests twice a week to monitor my condition.

I feel anxious about my future. I find it too difficult to cope with change due to the uncertain nature of cancer. I am taking anti depressants and often feel low and vulnerable.

Due to the fatigue and side effects of the chemotherapy I require to have someone with me at all times in case I fall ill.

I am also sick after chemotherapy sessions. This has required the doctor to be called at night on two occasions to administer anti sickness injections and I take regular anti sickness medication...

I sleep for approx two hours in the afternoon. The first two days after my treatment I spend in bed as getting out to go to the toilet is a struggle. The next four days I sit around the house as doing anything for more than ten minutes exhausts me.

I am required to stay away from places where there might be a chance of infections. Therefore I do not go out much due to my low immune system.

If my chemotherapy finishes I will be monitored for the first six months with twice weekly blood test, plus clinic visits in Charing Cross, London and Exeter hospital. I have been informed that my immune system will take months to return to normal and the fatigue will last for months. This is due to the weekly chemotherapy regime.

I have included my current medication list.

My husband, Trevor Coombs is acting as my carer both day and night and has written a letter of support of my appeal.

I have enclosed a letter of support from my Doctors Surgery Practice Manager, Mrs. Gillie Champion

I have also enclosed a letter of support from my specialist nurse at Charing Cross Hospital, Ms. Linda Dayal.

My doctor has previously submitted a DS1500

Should you wish to discuss any of the above information with me further, please feel free to phone me on the above telephone number.

Yours sincerely

I will let you know what their reply is.

Yes I am now exhausted after all the brain activity, but feel better for getting it on paper, even though as I said it does make hard reading.

27th November 2006

The early morning TV has been suspended due to the cricket. The Australians have opted not to play their matches during the night, therefore we have to suffer and become night owls. As with the British athletics team our cricket team are also allowing others to win. I think it is because as a nation we are such good losers!

I have spent most of the day on the sofa watching films, but don't worry I have had a sinus dressing done this morning!

I have also had a conversation with Linda about my incontinence problem. I did manage to ask the question 'is it the cancer coming back' Linda says it is as I have been told that my body is readjusting. I will be looked at when I go to London on Wednesday and then probably referred to an incontinence nurse. More to look forward too!

Even though I am writing about my waterworks problem I do find it embarrassing to talk about. I do feel like my body is failing me, but with all I am going through what do I expect.

Sally has just been in to see me. I think she is checking on me as her first question was 'have you phoned Linda'. But I'll let her off as it's nice to know she cares. She has also brought me a present, some incontinence pads and it's not even Christmas yet! I must get her something suitable for Christmas!

A few more days 2006

I phone the doctor as I have been feeling faint and breathless over the past few days and it's seems to be getting worse. Melissa answers the phone and says that Kieran will ring me back. Within minutes she phones back and says Kieran wants to see me in ½ an hour. Trevor takes me to the doctors as I am not driving now due to the fatigue and lack of concentration. I am greeted by Kieran who says 'you haven't got ill have you?' Kieran says I have malaise and fatigue. Well I been to Malaysia on holiday and I'm sure my symptoms aren't the same.

It's been another Charing Cross session. And only one to go but who's counting. Nothing to report on the journey up.

I appear to be developing a fan club at the hospital as Paul the bed manager is waving to me every time he passes. Doctor Tom inserts a cannula on the third attempt and I discuss with him my 'down below' problem. He thinks it is mechanical! So I suspect I will be off to the garage soon to have my sprocket fixed!

Paul is still waving.

Myooran comes to check in with me and is now talking about when my treatment is finished. This is good to hear but I won't believe it till it happens. He has also checked my scans to make sure there are no nodules in my brain. He'll be lucky as he will have to find a brain first. He asks if I have the CD's of my scans at home. I tell him that this is not primetime viewing in our house so no. Apparently the scan pictures stop half way down my chest. This must have been when the magician was sawing me in half! There are no nodules in my brain therefore Myooran also thinks my incontinence is mechanical. I wonder if they do body repairs on the side.

The chemo does not get any easier the more you have and I am not sure that you would ever get use to it. Just hearing the machine pumping the chemicals into me is enough to make me feel sick and I have several sick bowls by my bed just in case and the tiredness now starts within a couple of hours of the drip starting.

It is not easy going to the toilet with your arm attached to a drip when the stand the drip is on moves like a supermarket trolley. There is always one wheel that goes a different way to all the rest!

Paul is still waving and now smiling.

I see Linda before I leave and she asks me to get myself referred to the incontinence nurse in Exeter. She asks how this book is going and that Paul, the bed manager is hoping for a mention by name. So that's what all the waving was about! Well Paul you got your mention.

I do have something to report about the journey home. We have visited Tiverton service station so only 2 to go now. The excitement is almost too much for us to bear, but I'm sure we'll manage.

We arrive home at 5:00pm and I crawl into bed having already slept most of the car journey home. I set my alarm for the 4:00 am tablet place a sick bowl by the bed and I am soon asleep.

1ˢᵗ December 2006

The day has finally arrived. It's shower day. I have not had a shower for months (but I have washed so don't say it!) due to the sinus wound. Sally drops in some waterproof dressings with the message on it 'enjoy your shower'. I have even bought some chocolate smelling shower gel for the complete experience. At 3:15pm I get in the shower and allow the water to wash over me. You don't know how good the shower feels and the smell of the shower gel is heavenly. This is one of those little things that we take for granted until we can't have it and these little things mean so much to me at the moment.

I have my injection and the sinus wound dressed by Sally when she returns at 4:00pm. I ask her to refer me to the incontinence nurse. So another medical appointment to look forward to.

At 6:30pm the phone rings and it's Linda. This worries me as it's not working hours so I immediately assume that there is something wrong. She tells me she has read the latest episodes in this book and that there is just one thing. Have I upset someone? no she offers to write a letter of support for me to the Department of work and pensions. She says that I am doing really well. This means a lot to me, as she is someone who knows medically what I am going through.

It has touched me deeply that she rang when she should be relaxing. I do have to say that I have been amazed at the support that I have got from family and friends and there is no way that I could thank them all enough, but when I'm better I'll try.

2nd December 2006

Trevor is going to help Vicky tomorrow in her house, so he has rung Pat and asked her to wife sit. I am due to be dropped off at the nursery at 10:30ish and hubby will come to pick me up by 3:00.

Well I managed to behave at nursery I even took a packed lunch! But I didn't think much of playtime as I was too exhausted to go outside.

I have spent the rest of the day in bed as visiting is very tiring even if you don't do anything when you are there.

I am now becoming obsessed by the tablets that I take. I don't mind taking the prescribed drugs but when it comes to tablets that I have to choose to take I would prefer not to. I don't want to add any more chemicals to my body as I now feel the need to clean my system out of the poison that is in me. I have considered using our pressure washer but with all the holes in me I would look like the Trevi fountain, I would eat fresh food if I did not feel sick most of the time. Live yoghurt is out as I'm not allowed to eat it; maybe I'll try grass as cats use it to clean out fur balls!

I have my injection and dressing done and then settle down for the evening. The aches set in again which are stopping me from sleeping. I also feel restless again and I think that the frustration is back. I thought I had sorted that out. After 2 hours I revert to pain killers.

3rd *December 2006*

I keep waking up and thinking what I want to do in my garden. The pruning needs doing' I want to start a vegetable garden and sort out the waterfall to the pond. These will have to stay as thoughts as I am unable to get to the bottom of the garden which is on 3 levels and the steps are now too much.

Trevor is again helping Vicky but this time I am allowed 'home alone'. It's good to have some time alone although it is also a bit scary. Being alone gives me time to think and makes me feel not as I expected too. I have not been giving myself time to think in case it was too depressing but on the contrary it seems to be giving me some calm. It would be even better if I wasn't in my home where all the events of my life have happened. So if you have a solid, calm and peaceful place please let me know and I'll be there, alone.

I know I have mentioned my waterworks before well I now have another problem with water. We have lifted the front room carpet to find that the floor is wet. We have been told that our insurance company will not pay for the repairs so it's down to us. The reason I am mentioning this is we are taking it all in our stride. You see after all we have been going through this is minor. So if you have any funds for the lifeboat appeal donations will be gratefully accepted!

My vision now seems to be blurred. Not all the time and not necessarily when I am tired. I have checked my information and yes it is another side effect of the chemo. In fact checking the sheet I have or have had most of the side effects that go along with my chemo regime.

Well it would be a shame to leave any of the side effects out!

It's a good job that I decided not to drive a car a few weeks ago due to the fatigue and lack of concentration.

I have been out to a garden centre to buy a birthday card. I am now walking behind Trevor, no not because I have changed religion but because walking as fast as I did is not possible. Trevor has to slow down to walk beside me. I manage to buy a card and that is enough for me. Trevor would of liked a cup of coffee in the café but one look at the stairs and I am off to the tills.

We call in at my dad and step mums for coffee then home for me to rest and await the nurse. I am in bed early tonight and will be resting tomorrow so I make it to the theatre in the evening. So it's goodnight from me and a tablet at 4:00am.

4ᵗʰ December 2006

It's the day of the Vagina Monologues and Colleen has phoned to say she can't attend as she is ill. I phone around other friends but as its short notice no one can come. So Trevor to the rescue. He does not seem too happy about my suggestion of him wearing a dress!

Although I fully understand that my friends are busy, I would still have like to have gone with a female friend not only because it's a female play but also Trevor needs a rest from me and me from him. We are spending all day and night together apart from the occasional hour when he goes shopping. I think we both need some space, maybe when I am better.

I have spent most of the day in bed but this does not help much as I am still exhausted just by the car journey. I have decided not to sue the theatre as the Vagina Monologues were wonderful and I have not laughed so much for months. And yes Trevor found it funny as well. I have only just managed to sit through the whole performance and the walk back to the car is a real struggle. I ask Trevor to find a fish and chip shop as I have had no tea and it's now 10:00pm. Do the shops know who we are as every fish and chip shop we pull up at seems to be just shutting or have shut 5 minutes ago.

I am now tired, hungry and having a loud discussion with Trevor about how I need to eat before we get home or else I will only be fit to fall into bed without tea. This puts him under pressure and we end up in a 24hrs

Tesco superstore buying sandwiches. We call a truce on the drive home as we have both enjoyed the evening and don't want to spoil it but it's not us that is spoiling it, it's the cancer.

5th *December 2006*

A miracle has happened to me. Instead of being the super independent stubborn women that I am normally, I have decided to take care of myself. I have phoned Sally and asked her to come in and redo my dressing and take my FBC (KFC). This is unheard of but dragging myself down to the doctors surgery would be stupid as walking to the toilet is almost too far today. I know that this amount of fatigue was self inflicted but it was worth it.

I have phoned the doctors to let Melissa know that I won't be coming today. There is a bit of guilt about not making my appointment but I'm sure she will manage without me. I have also cancelled my appointment for tomorrow as I have made it the same time as my chemo; well I'm ill you know!

When Sally arrives even she is stunned that I rang, but is pleased that I made the call to her. I am repacked and this time she has taken blood out of me instead of injecting chemicals into me.

I have managed to stay in bed all day; well it wasn't difficult as my body was not willing to do anything else. I am not sure how you can spend the day in bed and still be tired, well I have successfully completed that task. The other thing that puzzles me is how you can be so tired and not be able to sleep; it must be the excitement of tomorrow's chemo!

6th December 2006

Of to meet my Exeter consultant at 9:20am and then to chemo.

Lizzie wishes to be mentioned here again as this time she thinks that you will imagine that we are 'best buddies'. I have also now been told by her that she will not be here for my final chemo on 20th December as she is on holiday. This is a real shame as she is one of the many people who have helped me so far and I am beginning to realise how hard it is to say goodbye to these people. This is not a usual medical relationship that I have with the staff that care for me. I think this is because with cancer I am in such a vulnerable position. There are times when I have not known whether I would live. The nursing staff seem able to acknowledge this without saying anything. There is an unspoken empathy that is held between not only the staff but also the other patients that I come into contact with and believe me it is very humbling.

I get home at 3:00pm and await Sally's arrival as one medical appointment is just not enough today! I am redressed again and Sally says that the wound is very nearly healed.

I am a little surprised to see Sally today as she said yesterday that she would be coming tomorrow but it may not be her! And I thought I was dazed and confused. Having witnessed Sally this week I have decided that my original plan to have my hair grow back blond is a mistake and I am now going for Trevor's plan of a blue rinse. I bet you can't guess what colour Sally's hair is?

I am dying (probably not the best word to use!) to talk to Sally about something that has been preying on my mind for about a week now, but it is not to do with anything medical and I am afraid of overstepping professional boundaries. So I say nothing.

I am not sleeping well at night as thoughts are again whizzing around in my head. I am also not able to decamp to the front room due to the underground swimming pool effect. Jen is busy building us an ark as I type.

My beta HCG (HSBC) is now 3.

7ᵗʰ *December 2006*

Another day in bed and I am feeling very sick today. I have taken all my anti-sickness tablets that I can and they are not working today. My sick bowl is within reach of my bed just in case I don't make it to the toilet.

Sadly the highlight of my day is the injection and dressing. I really must get a life! And guess what it's not Sally today even though she said it would be her!

My short term memory is playing its tricks again and I have

I'm still not sleeping during the night and neither is Trevor. We are both now down to about 4 hours sleep per night and believe me it is not enough. We are both grumpy and neither of us can explain the restlessness at night. We have tried watching TV till late, we have tried turning the TV off early, we have tried listening to the radio, we have tried having silence, in fact we have tried everything and nothing seems to be working. Do you think we might be stressed?

8ᵗʰ December 2006

I have managed to make it to the surgery to see Melissa for my blood test and yes she had managed without me but was surprised as one minute I was on the computer screen and the next minute I was wiped off. The problem was I was wiped out!

It's my dad's birthday today and I am going to see him even though it is only 2 days after chemo as I am getting more and more determined that the cancer is not going to run my life. Well that is apart from the fact that I need to be home by 3:30 to take the GCSF (GCSE) injection out of the fridge ready for my injection. So being the stubborn person I am Trevor's drives us to my dad's house. I manage to stay for an hour and that is enough.

I have just looked up to 4 paragraphs before this one and realised that I have stopped half way through a sentence. I am now laughing as I read I was mentioning my short term memory, if you wanted evidence of how bad it is, you now have it to be used against me at a later date!

What I should have written was; my short term memory is playing its tricks again and I have forgotten to make an appointment for my blood test tomorrow. I phone the surgery and luckily they can fit me in tomorrow morning. I really have had enough of needles but know that I just have to put up with it.

I have been planning ahead for Christmas and I know that you will be impressed when I tell you that I have bought the turkey and Christmas pudding. Unfortunately that's where the good part stops. The turkey is a ready rolled and stuffed breast crown because anything more difficult would be too much. The Christmas pudding is lost! When I say lost I mean I have put it somewhere safe and can't remember where that safe place is. More short term memory tricks. So we will be playing a new game at Christmas, hunt the pudding!

We both need a holiday but before we can book anywhere I have to check that it will be ok for me to go after my chemo has finished. We only want to go to the Forest of Dean, which is 2 hours away from our house, not Outer Mongolia and I am angry that I can't even book a few days away without having to ask first and have to organise how I have my blood tests done while I am away. I will put a holiday request form into Linda via the email and await her reply.

The holiday is also my first attempt at looking towards the future after chemo has finished.

The second attempt is to buy a massage table as I am a trained masseuse and this was to be my new career before I got cancer.

I am excited by the purchase of my new massage table but also scared at the same time as I have in the back of my mind all the time 'this could still all go wrong'.

I am still avoiding talking to Sally about the thoughts going round in my head.

At 2:00am I start to tell Trevor about what is going around in my head as we are both still awake. I now know where my calm place is and I am not sure what it is about but it's the solidness of a church. I don't think that it is anything to do with religion but more to do with a calm and peaceful atmosphere. Trevor is not so sure that it is not to do with religion as he can see why I might be looking for some kind of hope. He is willing to drive me to a church but does not want to come in. Due to my fatigue I will need someone with me so I will have to work on this one.

9ᵗʰ December 2006

I have decided that I will go shopping with Trevor today. The only problem is I appear to have wobbly legs. No I have not been drinking alcohol or started a cocaine habit. My legs just seem to have independent motion. By this I mean my hips and knees don't feel right and they are giving way when I try to walk. This is not happening all the time which makes me feel like I am auditioning for the ministry of silly walks. I'll push the trolley which can double as a Zimmer frame.

We go to a small supermarket and after 20mins I have had enough. I am getting ratty and have a go at Trevor due to the tiredness. On our return home I just fall into bed. Trevor has to bring all the shopping in, put it away and gets my lunch as doing anything else at the moment is not possible. So if the department of work and pensions is reading this, yes he is caring for me.

An artistic moment has come over me and I have started to paint. No not a wall, don't be silly even I know that I could not undertake decorating. I have placed a canvas on my easel as I can lose myself into a painting. It's going to be a moonlight seascape (I'll tell you this now so you know what it is when it's finished). There will be a reflection of the moon on the night sea with a few sailing boats. It feels like the right picture to paint as I am spending so much time awake in the night. If it turns out any good I will put a copy of it at the end of the book after the glossary. If it's rubbish you can use your imagination from the above description and make it look good in your mind for me.

Trevor is still trying to sort out the damp problem in the front room. This is frustrating for me as I would normally be helping him. I do wish that I was able to do more to help around the house and especially in the garden.

The sea in the painting looks good, however the sky is a different matter. The good thing about the type of paint that I use is you can paint over it and blend it in later. This is my plan. So you can see that my artistic talents are not working well.

The nurse arrives to inject and redress me, so I have to stop painting and realise how much paint I have over me. I'm sure I was supposed to put the paint on the canvas. My hands look like a playschool child's hands. I don't care as I am enjoying losing myself in the painting. I'm sure it will be a masterpiece given time!

I'm looking forward to another sleepless night, not! The aches have kicked in again and I am struggling with taking painkillers as its one tablet too many. The injections are also becoming too much again and if I felt I could get away with it I would tell everyone to go away and leave me alone. Every time that needle comes towards me I want to push it away and run in the other direction. I know that without any of this medical intervention I would die, there are just times when I have had enough.

10ᵗʰ *December 2006*

Yes I was right another sleepless night for both of us. The strange thing is that we are not that tired when we do wake up after about 4 – 5 hours sleep. I think we are becoming nocturnal. Who says we're stressed!

Its Archer's morning on the radio and Trevor is going out so I get the bed to myself.

I am glad that Trevor is going out as he has been banging nails for a few days now and I need some quiet. Don't get me wrong I am glad that he is sorting out the front room but I can't cope with a lot of noise or upheaval. You will laugh at the last comment when I tell you that the front room furniture is spread around every room in the house except the front room! It's like living in a furniture store. And yes I know that the sooner Trevor gets the work done the sooner the house will get back to normal but I'm going through my 'had enough' period.

I've sorted the sky out in my painting and it looks much better now you will be pleased to know!

The nurse arrives to inject and redress me and if you are fed up with me writing this then maybe you could understand why I am having my 'had enough'.

I have again spent most of the day in bed due to the wobbly legs and the 'had enough'.

My holiday request forms to Linda reads as follows:

I would like to request a holiday from the 22/1/07 to 26/1/07.
I would like to travel to Outer Mongolia (not really!) the Forest of Dean then.
I will be accompanied by Trevor (so at least there will be one sensible person there).
I will try and behave but can't make any promises.
How will I get my Thursday blood test done. (There is a hospital nearby)?
Will I be allowed in the swimming pool, sauna and steam room? Well someone's got to use them or it would be a waste!

It has just been emailed to Linda and I await the reply tomorrow. I have already made a note of the holiday accommodation phone number and downloaded the brochure onto my computer. Not that I'm keen to go!

11th December 2006

Linda is now my bestest friend ever! Because of the following reply:

Yes to all of the questions. You can go on holiday. You can use the sauna/steam room. By then you need once fortnightly blood tests. Any hospital can do this providing you give them the kits and instructions.

My holiday is now booked before you can say 'I'm ill you know'!

I have had my dressing done by Melissa this morning and have told her that I am having a day off tomorrow so she can cancel my appointment. I know that I should be having a dressing done but my wound has nearly healed and I am in my 'had enough' period. I get back into to the car and tell Trevor what I have done. He does not seem to be too happy with my decision, in fact he thinks that I have gone mad.

There is a loud discussion and when we get home he arranges for Sally to come in tomorrow and do the dressing. I am annoyed that he has done this but know that he is right, not that I'm going to tell him that!

While visiting my nephews, Caroline, my sister-in-law says that she has read this book and I should go on daytime TV as 'people like you' do that. She then realises what she has said and tries to dig herself out of the hole she has dropped into. I suggest to her that when you have fallen into a hole then it is not a good idea to grab a spade! We both laugh and decide that if this book did not already have a title then 'people like you' would be a good one. I will ask her at a later date when she has a few drinks what she means by people like you.

I've been out for a whole hour and I am knackered. Young children and cancer do not mix well, especially when you have got out of the young children routine. Having said this I would have missed not seeing them. So it's back to bed.

I am still in my 'had enough' period and don't want to go to Charing Cross this week for chemo. It just feels like on chemo too many. If they had given me the normal 6 maintenance sessions after my beta HCG got to 4 then I would have finished chemo by now. I do not want to be the chosen one who gets 8 chemo maintenance sessions. Even typing this I can taste the chemicals in my mouth and feel the cannula in my hand. I have not told Trevor how I feel about Charing Cross yet as he is still getting over me cancelling the first appointment and again I know that he will say I have to go and I know that he is right. I'll leave that surprise for him tomorrow!

12ᵗʰ December 2006

Oh yes Trevor is surprised and that is an understatement. He is struggling to understand why I would think like that when I only have 2 chemo's left. Well it does not matter how many chemo's there are left one more is too many and I don't want to go. I feel like a small child stamping my feet and saying leave me alone. I know and I think Trevor also knows that I will go to Charing Cross tomorrow but I can't help what I feel and I think I have every right to feel it.

Trevor thinks that my 'had enough' period is more to do with the cancer having ruled my life over the past few months and I will now have to manage without all the medical interventions I have had. I don't think that this is the reason I feel that I am just too tired to have one more thing done to me. Yes I am scared about what the future holds for me and there are questions that no one can answer. This includes will the cancer return after the chemo? I know that I should not be complaining as all the signs are positive that the cancer has gone, but after all that has happened to me over the past few months it is hard to believe that I might become cancer free.

The good news of the day is that the sinus wound has finally healed. It has only taken from the 24th September till now to heal. Sally is pleased, Trevor is pleased, I have had enough!

13th December 2006

Neither Trevor nor I have slept well but it's off to you Charing Cross (you knew I would, didn't you!). I focus on that this will be the last time that I will have to go to have chemo in London.

The mission of the day is to visit the last of the service stations. Exeter services being just up the road from us we decide to leave that to the journey home. So Bridgewater services here we come. Trevor takes a bit of talking into the quest but knows when to do as he is told (his theory for a long marriage is learning to say 'yes dear' and almost mean it! Well it's worked for the last 26 years!). The excitement of completing the penultimate service station was soon quashed by the realisation that we had been here before. Now this is the point where I can blame my short term memory, so what's Trevor's excuse?

We drive in and out the services and continue on to Charing Cross.

The journey is lightened by tuning into LBC radio. They are presenting a wants and found programme. One woman wants a square orange Sunbeam cooker with a lid which plugs into the electric. Another woman wants to know if anyone has a copy of a photo of her and Johnny Ray taken at a theatre in 1984! The best is saved to last! A man wants a Royal Doulton plate of Catherine Parr as his has fallen off the wall and smashed. Does this mean that history will have to be rewritten, will it now be Henry the eighth and his five merry wives of Windsor! The presenter has just collapsed in laughter as he has worked out that Catherine Parr was the wife who outlived Henry, well that was until she fell off the wall!

Wonders will never cease. Someone has a square orange Sunbeam cooker and is willing to give it away for free. I think it is one of those items that Auntie Ethel buys for you when you set up your first home. One of those gadgets that we all have in the back of our cupboards waiting for the day we can take it on Antiques

Road Show, still with it's original box and never been opened. This is another one of those moments that if it wasn't for my cancer we would have missed this moment and our lives would not have been complete.

Compared to the journey up waiting for my bed to become ready is uneventful.

Myooran is missing without trace, so I am visited by 2 other doctors who are now talking about what happens after the chemo has finished. I am still not quite able to believe that this nightmare is coming to an end. The doctor tells me that it is unlikely that the cancer will return and he is not expecting this to happen because I have reacted so well to the treatment. If the cancer does return there are plenty of other treatments available. I will continue to be tested by blood and urine tests and this will be monitored to make sure my Beta HCG (HSBC) levels do not raise again. My blurred eye sight should sort it's self out and I will start to feel my old self again by about the end of February. This last statement brings a groan from Trevor! I turn to the doctors and say 'have you met my husband!'

I tell them that I have booked my holiday so could my six week check up be after that, which is agreed. The doctor asks where we are going and I reply Outer Mongolia, he takes me seriously (he does not know me well) and tells me to stay out of the sun as I will get a nasty rash! This advice holds for the next year. So no sunbathing this year! I explain that we are going to the Forest of Dean and despite global warming we are not expecting sun at the end of January.

The chemo is not as bad as I thought it would be as I have now got my head around this is the last one at Charing Cross. I am asleep early in the evening and can't wait until the morning and I can leave for home for the last time.

14ᵗʰ December 2006

I have slept well and there is only a short while for the drip to run with the last of the chemo. By 9:30 it's all over and it's time for my massage session. This is bliss and relaxes me for the trip home.

Trevor appears to be upset because he has had his last fried breakfast in the restaurant. He has also left his mark on the restaurant staff. The cashier adds on the till Trevor's bacon, scrambled egg, tomatoes and fried bread, then asks if Trevor wants the tongs which he used to pick the fried bread up with that are now on his tray! And who says he's stressed.

My medication is up from pharmacy by 11:30 and it's just a visit to the Linda to ask what the follow up regime is in the way of blood tests. Linda explains to us how many tests I need to do. This would have been great if I could have remembered what she had said by the time I got to the car and after Trevor's episode with the tongs, we don't stand a chance. I'll email her later.

We tune into LBC radio again to hear the question and answer programme. This includes such topics as why do we have ear wax? Why do you have to go down so far for archaeological digs and where does all the earth come from? The answer is that ear wax stops infections and is an insect repellent. The earth worm is responsible for the amount of earth on top of archaeological ruins. So it's not only early morning TV where you can learn new concepts! I would like to thank LBC radio for putting my life into perspective.

I sleep for most of the way home and we both forget to visit Exeter services. We will save this exciting prospect for the six week check up.

I fall into bed and sleep for 2½ hours. Trevor is eating the lasagne that Becky has left for us which smells wonderful. I don't normally eat the night after chemo but the smell is too good. Unfortunately it did not smell quite as good on the way up 2 hours later! I set the alarm for the 1:10am tablet and drift back to sleep.

15ᵗʰ December 2006

Well I've managed to get to the surgery to have my bloods taken this morning. But don't worry because I am soon home and in bed again. I am resting today not only after the chemo but also because our friends Jen and Rob are coming to help move the furniture tonight so the front room carpet can be fitted tomorrow and to have a Chinese takeaway.

It is strange but I don't seem to be getting bored with all the time I spend in bed. Yes I am frustrated but I can always find something to do.

My massage table arrived yesterday and it is still in its bag. Trevor helps me put it up. Then will put it back into the bag and that's me finished for a while. So if you fancy coming and looking at the massage table but not getting on it I am charging £50 per hour for the experience!

I have had some more 'hand me ups' from Becky's friend, which is great as it will save me buying new clothes for my holiday. I have noticed that when I am given new clothes I look at them and think that I won't fit into them. My brain still thinks that I am the size I was before the cancer. This is the same for my hair. I still think I have hair on my head until I walk past a mirror, then I wonder who it is that I am looking at!

Sally comes to give me my injection. I have failed to tell you that I have finally talked to her about what was preying on my mind. I have decided that some things need to stay private and this is one of them, so sorry but this is one thing you will not find out about in this book.

The furniture is moved in the evening by Trevor and Rob and the Chinese takeaway eaten. The conversation as normal ends in laughter at Jen's long explanation of her Christmas plans. During this time I leave the room and put on the mini skirt that was in the 'hand me ups'. Well when I say mini shirt it looks more like a belt! I go back into the room and tell Jen I am off clubbing. If you can imagine a forty something bald woman in a belt you will realise how ridiculuos I look. But I do have legs now!

16ᵗʰ December 2006

The day starts well as Trevor has found the Christmas pudding. The day goes rapidly downhill from here. Trevor is making pesto and has decided to test the hand blender with his finger to make sure the blades are working properly. I think he is trying to get the sympathy vote.

I decide that Trevor needs to go to the hospital to get his finger dressed, and then I remember that I can't drive. So I call my dad to take him.

My dad arrives at the same time as the carpet fitter. The carpet fitter is confronted by a bald woman and a male with blood dripping down his finger. I welcome him in and reassure him that this is normal for our house. Luckily he stays and the carpet gets fitted.

One thing I have learnt is how to apply bandages which is lucky for Trevor.

Trevor arrives back with a bandaged finger and the possibility that his nail will come off. He now needs the finger redressed in 2 days so at least the nursing profession will still have one of my family to work on!

I have had the email back form Linda and I now need to have blood tests once a week. After the six week check up this will drop to once a fortnight which is different from what I thought. However it is much less testing than I thought so I'm going with it.

We attempt to put the furniture back into the front room during the afternoon but it proves too difficult with me having no energy and Trevor having a throbbing finger. So we soon give up and will wait for my brother to come tomorrow.

Another injection at 4:00pm and the flu like symptoms have started again this time with a running nose and aching limbs. So it's back to bed and another day over. Well not before the alarm is set for the 1:10am tablet. And who said life can be boring!

P.S. yes we did have pesto for tea! I made it!

17th December 2006

George, my nephew phones to say they are on their way. So we jump out of bed and get dressed just as the door bell rings. It's not long before I have a front room again.

Harry has been in our bedroom and runs into the front room and announces that my other hair is in the bedroom. He is looking at the hat on my head and thinking. I ask if he would like to see my head. He laughs and says yes. He laughs even more when I reveal my bald head. George continues to put the toy car he is making together. Harry asks why my hair has fallen out. So I tell him that I had to have some very special medicine which is different to the medicine that the doctor gives him and this is what made my hair fall out. I explain my hair loss in this way so that if he has medicine then he knows that his hair won't fall out. He tells me I must be a man. Well I don't think the chemo could do that to me. George has now decided that he wants to take a photo of my head on my brother's phone. I can only hope that this picture is deleted as my family would not be afraid to use it!

I rest for the next few hours as watching furniture being moved is enough for me. I have decided to attend a carol service in the evening which has a profound affect on me.

Another few day part 3

This week feels like it has been a bit of a blur. The thing that I was not going to tell you about is to do with finding my calm place in a church.

Well after the carol service again I think Trevor is right, in fact I can go now as far to say that I know Trevor is right and it is to do with religion. Cancer seems to have a way of turning my whole life upside down in ways that I did not expect.

The other major thing that has happened this week is that I have had my last chemo. Of course it was not without its problems, life could not be that simple could it? I have had a phone call from Kieran at 8:30am saying that my white blood count is raised (you know it's not good news when your doctor phones you at home that early in the morning).

He wants me to come in for a repeat blood test today. I tell him that I am going to hospital for my last chemo. He agrees to me carrying on with this plan but he will ring the hospital and tell them. I am worried that they will put off my last chemo. So I ring Linda to talk about the problem. She reassures me that the raised count is because of the GCSF (GCSE) injections. If there are any problems with them giving me the chemo I am to get them to ring her. I tell her that I will say that I know this hard woman in London who will sort them out. I offer to stand behind her as I feel that my bald head could help with the hard look!

My chemo is given with no need to call in the heavy mob. Then we wait for my last GCSF injection (GCSE) to take home. And we wait, and we wait. After an hour of waiting I am beginning to think that I have become so popular that the nursing staff can't bear to lose me. The nurse says that we can go home and come back tomorrow to get the injections. We don't need to be asked twice and leave before she can change her mind.

Trevor returns the next day to be told the injections arrived 2 mins after we left. Well we did not expect anything else.

I get into bed and feel a sharp pin in my neither regions. I feel down and can feel a small cut. The first thought is the cancer has spread. The second thought is this hurts. Trevor wants to take me to hospital now. Well I don't want to be a 'pain in the arse' (sorry but it had to be done!), so I decide to wait until the morning. I ring the doctors and get an appointment with the nurse.

I apologise to the nurse, as I am her first patient of the morning and she is going to have to look at my backside. She says that it is not to do with my cancer. I am prescribed some cream to use and told to keep an eye on it to make sure it does not get infected. Well I know I have lost a lot of weight but I am still not able to bend that far, so I'm not quite sure how I keep an eye on it but it could be fun trying!.

I seem to have arrived in limbo land. I have now to provide weekly blood tests and wait for my six week scan and check up. Six weeks seems a long time and I feel like I will want to hear the results of each blood test as soon as possible. Up to now I have not worried about what my beta HCG (HSBC) is doing as I am seeing doctors each week and they would tell me if there was a problem. Now I know that they will phone if there is a problem with my results but not seeing a doctor feels like I am alone. I'm sure that after a few weeks I will not be so worried. My routine of medical appointments has become such a big part of my life that I now feel insecure without them. Having said that, I am looking forward to getting some kind of normality back into my life. That is not me saying I am normal so don't get worried! I am normal for me and no one else!

I am really looking forward to my holiday in the Forest of Dean and Father Christmas will be here in a few days. This is a Christmas that I thought I might not see, so I am sure going to make the best of it as I am now chemically ready for Christmas. The tree is decorated, the presents are bought, the cards are sent and alcohol still tastes disgusting due to the chemo. So it's a teetotal Christmas for me.

I have found out how little alcohol I need to have to notice the taste. Becky and her partner Steve had taken us out for Sunday lunch. The carvery was nice, but the puddings look even nicer. I chose the one with Grande Marnier in it. Actually getting this pudding is another story. The waitress put our 3 chosen puddings on a tray. Becky held her card out to pay and I put my hands out to take the tray from the waitress. The waitress took one look at my headscarf and moved the tray away from me. I was not aware of the side effect that stops you from carrying trays! As I moved my hands closer towards the tray, she moved the tray further away. There is then the dance of the tray and the hands. I get to the point where I was contemplating a rugby tackle to get my pudding when she gave in and with a sigh of relief I got the puddings!!

I am hoping that someone will buy me a walking aid for Christmas as the wobbly leg syndrome seems to be getting worse. I am now finding it difficult to stand up. It does not matter how long I have been sitting down, my knees appear to have lost the ability to weight bear. I have to straighten myself up and get my balance before I move or the floor might hit me!

My fatigue is also worse I am wondering if my body knows that the chemo has finished and it is now breathing a sign of relief. I have had to keep going for the past fifteen weeks in which I have had fourteen sessions of chemo and now I can relax a bit more. My body is obviously going to make sure I do relax

23ʳᵈ *December 2006*

I have not mentioned early morning TV for a while. This is because I seem to be sleeping a bit better that was until this morning. Did you know that if you put the seat of your ride on mower lower to the ground it will go faster and you can compete in the lawn mower world championships!

My sight is not good today and it's nothing to do with the fog that is engulfing the country at the moment. Sometimes my vision is clear then the next minute my eyes seem like they have clouded over. It would make crossing the road a challenge if I could walk that far. Still, after all I have been through lately and survived, I am sure I will be run over by a bus.

I have had my penultimate injection today and have asked Sally if I can ceremonially burn the injection notes tomorrow. Apparently they have to keep my notes for their records. I feel that I need to mark the end of the treatment in some way but I am not sure how just yet. Setting fire to your district nurse instead of my medical notes is not a good option and anyway I have come to like her! Alcohol is out; maybe I could start my cocaine habit!

My hair is growing fast, by this I mean it is about 1cm long now and I can't do a thing with it! That will be because it is still too short. After all the worrying in the beginning about losing my hair, I am now excited and curious about how it will grow back. I look forward to the day I can run a brush through my hair again. I'm still not sure what colour it will grow back as I am told it could change colour as it grows. I don't care what it grows back like it will be just good enough to have hair again.

I have just had an idea. We will toast the end of my treatment with some of the gin and blackcurrant that Nina, my wig has been sat on for the past few months. I have just tested the drink and it tastes more of fruit juice than alcohol which is surprising as the gin has now been double fermented so will be about 50% proof. So its liqueurs all round tomorrow and a merry Christmas.

24ᵗʰ December 2006

I have planned a quiet day today; unfortunately no one else knows this!

Jen and Rob arrive first and leave when Simon, Caroline, George and Harry arrive.

Harry has written a letter to father Christmas asking for a real Gun (who does he want to shoot?) being only 5 years old he has spelt Gun wrong and I am sure given time my brother and sister in law will get use to the Gnu in their garden.

Sally arrives to give me my last injection and before she leaves Colleen and Garth arrive.

The significance of the last injection seems to get lost in the moment but we do manage to toast my last treatment with a dose of Nina. I am aware that this is a new stage in my cancer journey. I am now well into limbo land and I don't do 'wait and see' well. I want to know now if my beta HCG (HSBC) is going to rise and have my Scan today to make sure there is no more cancer. Yes I know that this is not possible but 6 weeks is a long wait.

By teatime I am exhausted and wonder how I will make it through Christmas day. So it's early bed and await Father Christmas (I would prefer George Clooney really, oh yes and Trevor!)

25th December 2006

Well I made it to Christmas. This was my personal goal that I set myself when the doctors told me I had cancer back in August. I have been determined whatever the prognosis that I would make it to Christmas. I feel very emotional having made my goal and at times during the day I am close to tears but as I don't want to spoil anyone's Christmas by crying. I hold back the tears.

We manage not to stuff ourselves at lunchtime and look forward to the Christmas pudding at teatime. We do not open our presents until Vicky arrives in the afternoon. I feel showered with presents this year. These include some garlic bulbs from Trevor. No not to ward off evil spirits (I think it may be to late for that!) but because I want to start a vegetable patch in our garden when I feel better and garlic is the main plant I have wanted to grow.

Then there's Jen and Rob's present. You just know it's not a box of Chocolates or some nice smelling bubble bath, it's a designer Beaver! You have to use the magnet pen to design how you would like you pubic hair to look with metal shavings. It even has pictures of pubic hair to choose from. Well it does not show the nude beaver that I am sporting at present, but that gives me time to design how I would like my hair to grow back. What a sweetie!

By 6 pm I am ready for bed but manage to stay up until both Becky and Vicky leave for their homes. I go to bed and I am asleep shortly. I sleep for about an hour then wake which is good as its Christmas and there are programmes that I want to watch on telly. By 10:30pm my eyes will not stay open anymore so off to the land of nod I go, well it's better than limbo land.

26th December 2006

Getting out of bed will not be accomplished today.

Trevor is starting to wind me up by suggesting that I should be getting more exercise. This is not the first time that he has mentioned this and I am not sure he realises what it is like living through cancer and a chemo regime. Does he not know that I would love to be doing more exercise; I would love to be putting in my vegetable patch or walking along a beach. He is asking me to do something that I would if I could but I can't. Does he not understand how frustrating this is for me? Well of course he doesn't unless I tell him as he has not developed telepathy yet! So I tell him and he now seems to understand.

It feels like the emotional rollercoaster has started again. I have no control again over what will happen to my cancer and I am not too fond of my visit to limbo land. I am trying not to let limbo land control my life too much though it is proving difficult when it is your life you are worrying about.

The return of another few days 2006

It's not that it's been Christmas that I haven't written but because the emotional rollercoaster has run off its tracks and has been freewheeling over some bumpy ground!

I have just realised that I have had a hysterectomy. Yes I know that was back in August but I've had a few things going on in my life and I'm ill you know! It's not that I want any more children (this is how I got here in the first place!) it's about being a woman and having my reproductive system removed. Most women have time to come to terms with the emotion implications of a hysterectomy before their operation. I had 3 hours. And that time was taken deciding whether to have full English or a continental. I am not sure how to explain how the operation has affected me but it feels very deep. Like a piece of me is missing (yes I know before you even think it!), the piece that makes men and women unique to their genders. That does not mean to say that I am not still a woman it's just that I have some bits missing. I don't feel whole. I also have the physical reminder of hot flushes daily. These are being made worse by my hair now growing. Before when the heat wave got to the top of my head the heat could escape because I had no hair. Now I have hair it keeps the heat in and I am sweating and clammy throughout the day and night. My sleep pattern includes the dance of the duvet which goes; duvet on, duvet off, duvet on, duvet off......

I am also emotionally now able to start reflecting on the past few months as I don't have so many medical appointments. It feels like I have been in a tornado and the debris is just beginning to fall back to earth. Not only is the debris falling to earth but I have been left alone to pick the mess up. I know that the last statement is not true as I am not alone because I have Trevor, my family and friends but this is the time when I feel like I need the support of the medical profession.

My physical health is also suffering. I thought that I would be starting to feel a bit better after the chemo had finished, however I am feeling worse. This has come as a shock to me.

My eyesight is a lot worse. My vision is blurred most of the time and on occasions anything more than 6 feet away it's difficult to see clearly. I am finding my sight problems distressing but know that it could be a while before this settles down. I can only hope it does settle down.

I have a tooth abscess which woke me up at 5am. I did what I had been told and phoned the duty doctor as an abscess is an infection. I explain to the doctor that I have cancer. He tells me to take 2 paracetamol and I should be alright. I have to explain again that I have cancer with little ability to fight infections due to having had 14 chemo sessions in 15 weeks (mother, eggs and sucking comes to mind here!). The doctor then says he will prescribe some antibiotics. After the cancer I am planning to train doctors!

I went into the city to change a pair of trousers. This for me is like running a marathon now. From the car park I had to climb 3 flights of stairs. When I finally get to the top I can go no further I rest against a wall as I am gasping for breath. I manage to change the trousers and buy a new swimming costume ready for my holiday. Then a slow walk back to the car which takes longer than the shopping and that is me for the day.

Trevor and I have looked after my nephews for 3 hours and I am exhausted after 2 hours. I know that I have got out of the routine of looking after young children but I now appreciate how much more difficult fighting cancer would be if I had small children to look after fulltime.

The computer battery has just shown me that it is low and I have asked Trevor if he could get me a new battery, if only my recovery both physical and emotional could be that easy!

A good bit of news; I have had an appointment to go and see an incontinence nurse. See life is not that bad! And even better there are 2 forms to be filled in before I attend. I have not filled in any forms for a few weeks now and was beginning to have withdrawal symptoms. So what have I got to be upset about!

1ˢᵗ January 2007
Happy New Year.

Well it might have been if I had no woken up with the abscess in my mouth now being the size of a golf ball. I guess the antibiotics have not worked. I phone Charing Cross at 6:30am as this is an infection and it hurts. Myooran is on call and says he will phone my local hospital to get me an appointment today as this cannot wait until after the bank holiday. He rings back and tells me that I am expected at the accident and emergency department at 9am.

So at 9am I am back in hospital. The doctor takes one look at my mouth and says the tooth will have to come out today. But you know it is not that simple! I have a full blood count first which takes an hour and then she wants to do the extraction in an operating theatre due to the risk of infection. So we go to the canteen and wait. And we wait. We then meet the doctor by chance and she has now booked a bed for me on a ward at 2pm just in case I need to stay over night. I only want my tooth out.

As we don't live far from the hospital we go home for 2 hours of which most of the time I am asleep. We return to the hospital at 2pm and I am admitted onto a ward. And we wait. At 5:30 Trevor goes to ask what is happening. The doctor arrives and tells us there have been 2 road traffic accidents and the theatres are full, so she will take my tooth out somewhere else in the hospital and use a nurse to assist her.

I am taken to a treatment room and covered in green cloths. The doctor puts on a gown, gloves and a mask as does the nurse. I am giving a pair of fetching green glasses as the lights are very strong. With my already blurred vision, green glasses and local anaesthetic I am now floating in pea soup.

I become a little concerned when the doctor asks me to breathe through my shoulders. This must be a new medical technique but try as I might I am not able to master it. I have to ask just as the doctor realises what she has asked me to do. Apparently I am to breathe through my nose and relax my shoulders. This technique I can do. Within a short while the offending tooth is out and I am stitched up and sent on home without having to return to my hospital bed.

I am exhausted and fall into bed feeling very sorry for myself. Then the tears begin and I am crying uncontrollably. This is another final straw. I just lay and cry. Trevor tries to comfort me but nothing is going to work until I have got the emotions out of my system. I am at last allowing myself to let go of all the feelings that I have had to hold in during my treatment. And I still don't want to die. I eventually fall asleep in a tear soaked pillow.

2nd *January 2007*

Trevor has made an appointment for me to go and talk to Gillie at the doctors this afternoon after last night. So I spend the time until my appointment lying around the house. When I get to see Gillie she asks me how do you eat an elephant? This stuns me a bit and I don't know how or what to reply. She explains that you have it eat an elephant in bite size chunks and that is how I need to live at the moment. I need to set goals and give myself back some structure which is now missing from my life since all my medical appointments have stopped. I also need to set realistic goals each day. I only want to bake a cake and prune the roses I tell her. I don't think this is too much to do. I do understand what she means but I want to do everything that I could do before my cancer and I want to do it now!

I feel a bit lighter after talking to Gillie even though this is the small kind of thing that Trevor had told me last night. It's just good to hear it from someone who is not so closely involved with me.

Tomorrow if I'm really good I will bake a cake in the afternoon.

3rd *January 2007*

Before cake making there is my Wednesday blood test with Melissa. I have already had blood taken on Monday from my best vein so today will be my second best veins turn. The only problem is that this vein has decided to give blood one drip at a time. Neither Melissa nor I are too impressed by this and give up at a half full bottle of blood. We both hope this will be enough for the beta HCG test. There is no way that I am going to let her stick another needle in me and she doesn't even ask.

I have decided to make a carrot and pineapple cake as this will have 2 of the 5 recommended fruit and veg. per day and is therefore a healthy option! Grating the carrots exhausts me and once the cake is in the oven I sit on the sofa and rest. After 40 mins the cake is baked and I feel a sense of satisfaction. I have managed one of my goals. Tomorrow I will prune a rose. By Easter I will climb Mount Everest (only joking!).

I sleep for a while at teatime as my next goal is to visit my pantomime friends who are rehearsing tonight. I am woken by a phone call from Myooran who wants to know how I am. I discuss with him my eye sight. He tells me it will take about 3 to6 months for the chemo drugs to wear off completely. Well at least he thinks I will live this long! My beta HCG test is very positive with my latest test result being 3. We talk about my preferred date to return to Charing Cross hospital for my 6 week check-up. I would like the 29th January but Myooran would like the 5th February as he is on holiday the week before and would like to see me again (see I knew they would miss me at the hospital when my chemo had finished!). Myooran tells me it is because I am unusual and unique. I'm sure this must be a compliment!

I manage a quick visit to the Panto in the evening. It is good to see everyone trying to work out if they should be coming on stage right or left and forgetting their lines. I remember this well from last year when I was the queen of Whitstonia in Sleeping Beauty. It also makes me feel sad as I want to be on stage with them but I'm glad I made the effort to get there.

4th January 2007

I start this morning with an eye test at the doctors. Drops are put into my eyes to dilate the pupils. So now not only do I have blurred vision but I can't stand the light. This will rectify itself in about 2 hours and I do look very cool in sunglasses in January! I could always take my hat off and give people the full effect with my bald head but this may well be too much for the general public.

After lunch I prune a rose. That's 2 chunks of elephant in 2 days, before the month is out elephants will be an endangered species!

Well after eating 2 elephant chunks I'm tired. So would you be as the skin is very tough and the abscess makes my mouth hurts.

I'm fit for nothing the rest of the day which is not a problem as I have nothing to do for the rest of the day.

I go to bed having taken several pain killers and rinse my mouth with a wonderful salt solution.

5th January 2007

I am woken by the phone, actually this is not the first time I have been awake. I needed to refill with pain killers during the night. The phone call is from a publishing house who is interested in helping me let loose this book on the general public. This lifts my spirits. It's amazing how different I feel now compared to the beginning of the week.

The second phone call of the morning is from my consultant in London's secretary. The date has been set for my six week check after chemo. It will be 5th February. So now I have something to aim for. That means that I will finish writing this on the 6th February. That's a relief!

I have decided to start to write the questions that I want to ask on the 5th in my diary as I will never remember them tomorrow let alone in a few weeks time. I want to know when I can start HRT treatment to stop the hot flushes and will my cancer be cased as in remission or will I be cured if my Beta HCG remains low. I'm sure I will think of more question in the coming weeks.

I am in two minds about starting HRT as this is putting another chemical into my body and I'm not sure that I am ready for this yet. I would like to give my body a rest to recover.

Next it's off for a massage, which is the first one since my chemo has finished. So this time I don't feel sick, but don't get too excited my mouth hurts and I have to use extra towels to support my cheeks when I lay on the table on my front. I am hoping that when I have my next massage there will be nothing wrong and I can have a massage where I can just relax.

I'm sure my mouth is hurting more today and I only hope that the infection has gone. The pain is into my ear up to my eye socket and down the side of my nose. It still feels like the final straw as I am suppose to be recovering from the cancer now not having to fight another infection.

Today's elephant chunk is to go shopping with Trevor. A quick whirl around a supermarket is enough for me as its pain killer time again. I've checked the shelves of the supermarket and there are no tins of elephant chunks.

I have decided to replace the metaphor of the elephant with one of my own which is true. We have recently tried to grow mushrooms in a box. After keeping the mushrooms at the exact temperature suggested in the instruction for weeks with no sign of any baby mushrooms appearing we throw the box into the garden and gave up hope. Yesterday I found the box under the garden table in winter temperatures and guess what, there are now baby mushrooms appearing. So when you think there is no hope don't give up as you may come up smelling of mushrooms. You just need to find the right conditions, start as a small spore and nurture yourself until you grow.

6th *January 2007*

My mouth does not hurt as much today, hurray! I do feel very tired but I am not going to push myself to do anything because I'm ill you know.

The mushrooms are getting bigger by the minute, well it seems like that. Do you think I could front an early morning TV show on Zen and the art of mushroom cultivation or is this one step too far? I think the latter!

I have spent most of the day lying on the sofa and I'm proud of it! I am even not going to write anything more now so goodnight until tomorrow.

7th *January 2007*

This may not seem much to you but I have just shampooed my hair for the first time. It has grown enough to make using shampoo worth while. I have used baby shampoo as my hair is very soft and I don't want to damage my new growth as it is very precious to me.

I want to tell everyone I meet that I have washed my hair but I don't think that your average person would understand and the men in the white coats might be sent to get me! So I go around with a smile on my face like the cat that has got the cream. Before you know it I will be wearing a pink ribbon in my hair.

Everyday seems to be a tired day at present. I went out for 2 hours this morning and that's me for the day. I have slept for an hour in the afternoon and my mushroom for today is to cook the Sunday lunch.

I have managed to cook Sunday lunch using my excellent time management skills. These enable me to cook in stages with rests in between. I am expecting lunch to have finished cooking by June!

Although I have cooked the Sunday lunch, dishing it up is one step to far so that will be Trevor's job (this was calculated in my time management plan honest!).

So its food then off to bed for me after what has been a momentous day.

8ᵗʰ January 2007

I am certainly paying for all the excitement of yesterday. Getting out of bed this morning is not going to happen. I should explain what it feels like when getting out of bed is not possible. My body feels heavy and lifeless. My muscles ache and just the thought of moving is beyond me. It's not that I want to stay in bed as I have a life that is waiting for me to join it, but it will just have to wait until I am ready.

The afternoon is taken up by a visit from Jonny, the vicar of Digby. I find this very comforting and yes I will admit it is to do with religion!

I am determined to get out today so Trevor and I go to two shops. These are next to each other and I don't walk far. The prospect of a 3rd shop is not a good one so I ask to go home. Well at least it was a small mushroom!

I am counting down the days to our holiday. This cannot come too soon and I have mentally packed my suitcase several times already.

Writing about my holiday reminds me that I have to arrange a blood test on the Wednesday that we are away. I contact the local hospital to the holiday park. They have never heard of a Beta HCG test and seem a bit reluctant to take my blood. I reassure them that I have the test kit, I can talk them through the test, point out where my best vein is, and in fact if they give me the needle I could probably perform the test myself. This seems to convince the sister in the emergency department that this will not be as difficult as she thinks. She has not met me yet so I will not shatter her dream yet!

13ᵗʰ *January 2007*

Where did the last five days go? Days just seem to blur into each other. There are times when I only know which day it is by the medical appointment I have to attend.

The mushrooms have grown so much that we will be having steak and our own mushrooms for tea.

The holiday is getting ever closer, and I just hope that neither of us get ill before next Friday.

I am finding it difficult to look forward without fearing the worst (as you can see from the last paragraph). I can manage planning ahead about two days, but beyond that there appears to be a block that comes up in my head that won't let me think about the future. It's not that I don't think that there will be a future for me, it's that I am now use to living for today because who knows what will happen tomorrow. I have made my New Year resolution, which is to live for the rest of my life.

Trevor and I have been having a disagreement about my recovery. He thinks that I should be doing more towards getting fit. Becky thinks I should be going to aqua aerobics. If I went to aqua aerobics with my current fatigue levels I would drown! Both of them don't seem to understand just what my body and mind has been through. I think they feel that I have finished my chemo and should be better now. I would like to be better by now, we are all thinking in the same direction. It's just that my body needs time to catch up with everything. Part of me wants to march them down to the doctors and let him tell them that it is a 3-6 month recovery period, but I will tell them myself. I'm not sure how Trevor has missed the doctors talking about my recovery, but as he has also been under a lot of stress I can see how this has happened. I will talk to him later when I have calmed down, but in the mean time I am off to bed.

14th January 2007

I am drinking cranberry juice as I have developed cystitis. I have been taking tablets brought at the chemist as it is Sunday. I will have to make a doctors appointment tomorrow as the tablets are not working and I am going on holiday on Friday and I will be well! I think that it must be my lack of immune system that makes any infection take hold and need stronger medication than you can buy. I'm sure that I must have got my season ticket to the doctor's surgery by now and it is only a matter of time before they name a chair after me!

I have managed to complete a small amount of gardening this morning. By this I mean I have directed Trevor as to how to prune a tree and which way to lay stones in the fish pond. I did do about five minutes of sweeping the decking and that's it for me. I do have a sense of achievement as this is more than I could have done a month ago, but wish I could do more.

Trevor has today booked us into the visitor's accommodation at Hammersmith hospital on the 4th February. He certainly knows how to show me a good time! There is no way that I could manage to travel up and back to London in one day especially if I have to leave early in the morning. So we will travel up on Sunday and be there ready for Monday. I don't think that this will make the day less stressful, but at least I will be awake to ask the questions I want too.

My sister in law is in hospital having her appendix out, and wants to add a chapter to this book called 'I'm ill too'. I've told her I will put it in the appendix at the back of the book!

I have inspected her food tray only to find that it does not matter which hospital you are in there is always a story about the food. Caroline has ordered soup and a piece of fruit, so why do they send this on a tray with a cover. The soup and fruit are not under the cover; in fact nothing is under the cover! Just an empty tray, with the soup and fruit beside it. Is it me?

24th January 2007

I have to apologise at this point as I have failed to keep the writing together, but I am ill you know! I have become a relapsed cancer addict you see. Yes the cancer is back and I have had to take some time to get my head together before I could put fingers to keyboard again. So I will now attempt to bring you up to speed with my life.

I have had an appointment with the incontinence nurse. She has diagnosed a stressed bladder, or in her words my bladder has taken umbrage! It is not the only part of my body that has done this. Apparently a bladder is suppose to be soft and elastic, well not mine! My bladder has decided to throw a strop and has gone solid. Therefore it just wants to empty itself all the time. I am now in the process of retraining my bladder, no not sit and stay, but wait.

Then my world begins to turn on its head. My beta HCG is 6 which is above normal. This had better be just a glitch as it is a few days to our holiday. Having said this in the back of my mind I know that something is wrong.

I try to pretend that everything will be alright which I maintain until the evening. Then the tears start and I feel like I am back at the beginning again. I'm crying and I don't want to die. I curl up in bed and sob into the pillow; nothing comes close to comforting me. I know the cancer is back without having anymore blood test, as my body is changing again. By this I mean that my breasts are getting sore again with is due to the rise in HCG in my blood.

After a good cry it's time to move on and get myself sorted. It appears that once I have had my crying time then I am stronger and able to start taking some control over myself again.

Its holiday time and we set off in the morning knowing that I have to make a phone call to check my HCG levels at lunch time. And then as if by magic it's lunch time. I phone to be told that my HCG reading is now 22, and there is a meeting going on now to discuss what the next steps should be. I tell them that I will be phone back in 2 hours as the only place that I can pick up a mobile phone signal at the holiday accommodation is standing next to the telephone box!, that's modern technology for you!

After the longest 2 hours ever reported I make the call to be told that there is a bed booked for me in six days time at Charing Cross hospital. I reply that I am on holiday and my friends are coming to stay. Which now seems silly, of course my health comes first. It's just that we have both been looking forward to our holiday so much and now we are going to have to cut it short for me to go back into hospital.

Nothing is going to stop the holiday time we have got, so after all the phone calls are made to family and friends we are determined to have a good time. It's just nice being somewhere else other than where all medical interventions in my life happen. so holiday we do as it would be a waste not to use the swimming pool, Jacuzzi, steam room and sauna. I still feel too unwell to use the gym (well that's my excuse and I'm ill you know!).

25ᵗʰ *January 2007*

All too soon the holiday is over and I go straight to Charing Cross Hospital with out passing go and or collecting £200 pounds.

Within minutes of entering the hospital I am in the nuclear medicine department I am being prepared for my first test. You just know it's not going to be nice when the injection that they want to insert into your arm comes in a lead container! I am injected and told to return in 2 hours for a blood test to be followed by a further blood test 2 hours after that. So a quiet day is not in store for me.

Next is the MRI scan. I am laid on a sliding table which has been designed for people of restricted weight. Not being of restricted weight myself this proves to be a little uncomfortable to say the least. Just to add to my fun and enjoyment of the experience my head is clammed to the table and I am inserted into what seems like a Smartie tube. This sends me back to my childhood and I remember watching Joe 90, who sat in a strange machine which spin around him and gave him super powers. I am sure that my super powers will be great and enable me to solve the problems of mankind! The lottery numbers could take a little longer!

After 40 mins in the MRI I'm spun out and it's off back to nuclear medicine to have the first lot of blood taken. Then there's no time to rest for the wicked and off for a CAT scan, but I don't have a cat with me, in fact I don't have a pet cat at all! The staff don't seem to mind the lack of cat and scan me anyway! I am injected during the scan with a chemical which first makes me feel hot, then makes me feel like I am wetting myself, which the nurse tells me is normal, does she know about my incontinence problem? I won't ask!

Next up to the ward to check in. After waiting for a lift to take me up to the 6th floor I just have time to find a nurse to show me to my bed, and then its time for my ultrasound scan, so back to the lifts, down to the first floor and return to the x-ray department. I am hungry and have just remembered that I should be drinking lots of water ready for the scan. I send Trevor to the water dispenser where there is a lack of cups. I could just put my mouth under the tap but a cup would be better, so the receptionist goes off to track down some cups and arrives back 5 mins later with one cup. Has the health service got a policy on cup sharing as by now there are other people who also need to drink water, well they are not sharing my cup! Off goes the receptionist again, maybe she is the cup monitor of the day!

After several very quickly downed cups of water I need a wee! Luckily my name is called before the incontinence starts. So here I am again covered with cold gel and the ultrasound technician moving the hand held scanner around my stomach area. I can see the screen which reminds me of a snow storm. This appears to be a problem as that is all there is a snow storm! The technician is going pale and beginning to match the screen in complexion. This is worrying as I am watching him and watching the screen and nothing is happening. The hand held scanner in now moving ever more erratically around my stomach and I really do need a wee. Then it hits me and I say "do you know that I have had a hysterectomy" the colour immediately returned to his face and he says "that's why I can't find the uterus" "well don't look for the ovaries either, try scanning a jar as I don't have any of these either" I tell him. The male pride then kicks in and he then decides to stop looking for anything else and does not perform the internal scan. I just want a wee and no one is going to stop me.

At the speed of light I'm off to the toilet, what a relief!! And to think that I did not need to drink all that water anyway!

Back on the ward I eventually get to lie down for a while, however don't get too excited as its blood test time again so back to nuclear medicine. By teatime I feel like I have run a marathon.

I am visited by Myooran who tells me that he thinks I will be having some more chemo. Well lucky me! The chemo will be a different regime which is fortnightly, but will all be in London (we'll see about that!). The best bit of news is tomorrow I get to experience a lumbar puncture. They will be testing my spinal fluid to see if any of the cancer cells have made it to my brain. Not a lot gets to my brain at the best of times, so this is unlikely! I have heard of this procedure and nothing that I have been told about a lumbar puncture is good. So I'm going to forget about it for tonight. Myooran says that they can see a 7mm lesion on my lung which was on the first scan I had, but has not changed shape. This could be the rogue cancer cells but they cannot be sure. The cancer is still Choroicarsomia and has not become lung cancer, so the prognosis is still good. This gives me hope again, which I really need at this time.

Trevor leaves for his accommodation and I settle down to sleep. Trying to make sense of what is happening is just too difficult. Sayings like 'it can only happen to me' come to mind, but I know that's not true as I'm on a cancer ward and it's happened to others too.

26*th* January 2007

A morning of resting on my bed, and an afternoon of being restless on my bed! Doctor Tom has the pleasure of performing my lumbar puncture. I even get to have the procedure on my bed with the curtain drawn round, so swearing is out! At 3 o'clock it's time. Doctor Tom has done his warming up exercises and he's going in. I am curled up on my bed lying, on my side trying to touch my knees on my chin. Being a middle aged woman this does not come naturally. Doctor Tom suggests that Trevor stays to give me some support. I know from the last statement that this will not be easy. I am given some local anaesthetic into my back, which stings then goes numb. Then I can feel the needle being pushed into my spine. I am gripping the side of the mattress with both hands and may well rip the material at any point. Trevor looks at me trying to not swear and says "I can't feel a thing" at this point his head may come off! But it does distract me for a while. At last it's over. Well when I say over I now have to lie on my back for the next six hours and not move as I may feel faint due to the fluid that has been removed from my spine.

Dinner arrives and I try to work out how I am going to eat roast chicken lying on my back. I could just scoop it into my mouth as the plate is at the same level as my mouth. I am certainly not going to ask Trevor to feed me, so I turn on my side and put the food into my mouth carefully!

Next it's bed pan time. I ring the bell in plenty of time and position myself ready. Then my mobile phone bleeps, it's a message from Jen. As I know that the removal of a bed pan can take a while I decide to reply while still balancing on the pan. I am wrong; half way through my text the nurse arrives to remove the bedpan. I put my phone down beside me and start to shuffle of the pan. This does not go to plan. I fall off the pan onto the phone which sends half a text message to Jen and covers the bed in urine! After a bed change which involved me having to move around the bed I text Jen back with the rest of the message and explain that I fell off a bed pan and that's why she only got half a message!

27ʰ January 2007

Release day. I am allowed home till Monday when I have to return to be nuked. That gives me 1 ½ days at home and 2 nights in my own bed.

The thought of another service station lunch is too much, so we broaden our horizons, and visit Ikea for meatballs. I manage to walk half way around the store after lunch and that's enough for me. I think that this is the first time I would have been up for saying yes to a wheelchair, but opt to leave the store instead, having brought only half the items I wanted. It's home and straight to bed for me and that's where I am going to stay.

My Beta HCG is now 203 and counting

28th January 2007

We are having a quiet day before returning to Charing Cross tomorrow.

Trevor has got himself into a state about getting up early in the morning and is sure he won't sleep, so that a sure thing now. I have to take 10 tablets at 8pm and another 10 at 6am. I have failed to ask what the tablets are for, but it is not long after taking the first 10 that I work it out! They are steroids and I am now capable of running the London and New York marathon before morning.

29ᵗʰ January 2007

I retire to the front room at 3:30am to watch early morning TV. I have now acquired the new skills of cabinet building and can cooked goat curry!

Trevor is attempting to sleep. This is not going well and he is getting grumpier by the minute. I have decided to stay out of his way just in case he falls asleep by mistake.

We leave at 6:30am (yes there is such a time!), stop for 15 minutes on the way and get to London by 10:45am.

I am still on my marathon run having taken the second lot of steroids. After a quick visit to clinic, I'm off for my first chemo. This one is called PAC-E.

Linda is going to give me my chemo and the first injection is a large dose of piriton. Within a short while my eyes are closed. Then I'm awake again, however I appear to have lost the ability to speak straight and ask Linda for the results of my scat can (CAT scan)! She asks me if this was the test to see how scatty I am. She's a cruel woman taking advantage of a person on chemo!

Trevor has gone to pharmacy to get my tablets and returns without my GCSF injection which have not been requested. A doctor is tracked down to write a prescription and this is passed to pharmacy. All goes well to this point.

Trevor	Are my wives injections are ready yet?
Pharmacist	Are you Mr. Goff.
Trevor	No
Pharmacist	Is your wife called Francesca.
Trevor	No, but that is my wife's birth date.
Pharmacist	I'll give you the injections and sort the rest later

Has he remarried without telling me? Has he changed my name while I was asleep?

After a good nuking I'm on my way home. Again sleep comes soon and I wake as we arrive home at 10pm. We both fall into bed after another exhausting day.

Beta HCG 273

1ˢᵗ *February 2007*

The side effect of the chemo has started and I can report that moving hurts. I have tried paracetamol and ibuprofen but it's not touching the pain. I phone Charing Cross and speak to Doctor Tim. He suggests I get some tramadol from my doctor.

Prescription sorted, tablets taken and I'm off the planet! Floating around the ceiling I have no pain and no grasp on reality. It's a great feeling and I'm going with it. Does this mean I am now a drug addict?

I don't feel the GCFS injection going into my arm; in fact I can't feel anything. That reminds me I can't feel the top of my fingers or toes. This is called peripheral neuropathy (impressed or what) I can only describe the feeling as having been playing in the snow till you can't feel your finger tips with added tingling. This does make picking up small items rather difficult and typing has become interesting, as I am not sure whether I have pressed the keyboard or not!

The night brings unexpected highs. I wake at about 2:00am and ask Trevor to go and check downstairs as I am convinced that we have a burglar. He does not want to go downstairs and tries to calm me. This makes me even more determined that he should stop being a wimp and go and check. I eventually fall back to sleep. In the morning Trevor tells me about my nights exploits and we both fall about laughing. It may have taken a while for him to check downstairs as we live in a bungalow!

I have a new theory which I feel I should share with you. The cancer is not going to kill me, but the oncoming bus will. I will explain.

I will not be able to see the bus coming due to my eye sight,
I will not be able to hear the bus coming due to the tinnitus,
I will not be able to run out the way of the bus due to the fatigue,
Therefore my bus theory wins!

I have emailed Linda with the following request;

Since coming off of my anti depressants my sex life has suffered but the use of steroids is a near substitute so could I please have some extra steroids for medical use?

It is not long before Linda rings laughing to tell me that she does not think that her role can run to extra steroids to enhance my sex life. I suggest to her that as my specialist nurse she should be seeing not only to my physical needs, but also my emotional needs. You just can't get the nursing staff these days!

3ʳᵈ *February 2007*

It's Panto time. Oh no it's not, oh yes it is! I have really missed not being in the Whitestone pantomime this year and have very mixed feelings about going to watch it. I sit in the audience and wish I was on stage, but I do know that I would have managed about 2 minutes on stage, so I would not have been much of an actor this year. Here's hoping for next year. Having said this I did thoroughly enjoy the Panto and would not have missed it for the world.

Trevor has decided that he should build me a kennel at the bottom of the garden as he says that 'people like me' should not be allowed in the house. He is sure that the planning permission will be no problem as he is employed by the government as my carer! He has offered to install heating in the kennel as I am ill you know. What would I do without him?

Beta HCG 482

5ᵗʰ *February 2007*

I'm not feeling very well today. I can't quite say what is wrong with me I just know I'm not right. So I make an appointment with our doctor. Kieran takes a blood test and gives me a prescription of antibiotics. He says he will phone me tomorrow with the results of the blood test and will tell me if I need to take the tablets. I am also worried about Kieran, our doctor, as he agrees with Trevor about the kennel and could call around at anytime to help build it!

By 2am I am sat on the edge of the bed crying, as I really do feel very ill now. Trevor phones the duty doctor who says he will see me if I go into the hospital. So off we go in the middle of the night. When we arrive Jen is on duty at the hospital. It's good to see a friendly face. The doctor calls me in and says that I should wait until the morning to find out the results of the blood test. But I don't feel well, in fact I'm too ill to argue and I go home again.

6ᵗʰ *February 2007*

I lie in bed and feel sorry for myself. I cancel the plans to go and see Colleen and stay in bed. Colleen decides that she will come to see me instead, so I get out of bed and feel a bit better while she is here. By 2:00pm I am ready for bed again. As soon as my head hits the pillow I'm asleep. I am woken by the phone ringing. It's Melissa from the doctor's surgery saying that I need to phone Linda now as my white blood count is 1.8, which is very low. I told them I was ill! I bleep Linda who asks me to take my temperature. It's 38.1c. She says that she will arrange for me to go into my local hospital as I am ill, well what a surprise! I'm in hospital and admitted into an isolation room within an hour. So now they believe me.

Trevor leaves for home when he feels I am safe as he is also unwell. The doctor takes more blood tests. At 11pm I am taken in a wheelchair to have an x-ray. At 11:30 I am put on an intravenous antibiotic drip and also given oral antibiotics. My temperature is monitored through the night as it is rising fast, as is my pulse rate. My blood pressure is dropping. So sleep in not much of an option tonight.

7ᵗʰ *February 2007*

Trevor arrives at 9:00am and says that they have told him that I have had a bad night. Well are you surprised! By now my temperature is

39c, my pulse 117 and my blood pressure going down. It's not going well!

By lunch time I have got to 39.5c and the nurses are looking worried. I am not concerned as I am not sure what is going on anymore, and staring at the ceiling has become an art.

I am pumped full of more antibiotics and by teatime my temperature is starting to drop. I begin to realise what is happening to me which shows that I am getting better. I realise that I am shut in one room with a commode. Everyone who enters is wearing aprons and any visitors I have must report to reception before they see me. See I am ill.

I just drift through the rest of the day and get a good nights sleep.

8ᵗʰ February 2007

I am much better today, in fact by the afternoon I can have the door open of my cell. Although I'm not allowed out of the door yet. I am beginning to eat again and the doctors are pleased with my progress. I am even told that I my get parole tomorrow if I'm good. Apparently I became neutropenic, which means my immune system collapsed. See I was very very ill!

9th *February 2007*

I have been given parole and been allowed out of the cell and on to the main ward. I don't have the drip anymore, just oral antibiotics. I am up and about today and have a promise that I can return home tomorrow.

In the evening I lie in bed and wait for my 11:00pm tablets. It gives me the opportunity of watching T.V. Well I'm stunned; one of the channels is showing a programme called how to be a porn star. Only I can find pornography on a hospital T.V! I haven't had any steroids and frankly I don't feel like sex just at the moment; however I do try to laugh quietly into my pillow. I'll mention what I have found tomorrow to the staff as for once I find myself speechless!

Beta HCG 148

12th *February 2007*

After an early morning visit to the hospital to have my FBC (KFC) blood count taken to see if I can have chemo tomorrow I have a conversation by phone with Linda. I update her on the comings and goings of last week and tell her that I have made a decision that

I would like a line put into my arm so I don't have to have a cannula inserted each time I am having chemo or any other drugs injected into me. I am not sure that I have any veins left so becoming a cocaine addict is out for the time being! She agrees and says that I can have a picket line, well that's what I think she called it. She will try and sort this out when I come to Charing Cross tomorrow.

I have now looked on the internet and it's a Picc line not a picket line. Well I was close! The line is inserted into my arm just below the elbow and threaded into a vein, up my arm and finishes just beside my heart. So something to look forward to then! Can my life get anymore exciting? I wish I hadn't asked for a line now, but I know it will make life easier!

I contact Charing Cross at 4pm to be told that my blood levels are fine and I can have Chemo tomorrow which is a relief and a pain at the same time. I am caught between wanting to have the chemo done and having a rest after the trials and tribulations of last week. Its steroid night and I wouldn't want to miss the high, so opt for the chemo. At 10pm I start the ride by taking the first 10 steroid tablets. That makes 15 tablets to take in one go with all the other medication I am on, so I will either be kept awake by the effects of the steroids or be visiting the toilet all night due to the amount of water needed to take all the tablets!

13th February 2007

4:13am and it's a combination of the toilet and the steroids. I have managed to sleep a bit, but now I am awake I keep getting the giggles. You see my mind has gone into overload and I think the most stupid things, for example; I am sure that Trevor is lying next to me awake, so I turn to see if his eyes are open. This would have been an excellent test to see if he was awake apart from on small technical point, it's the middle of the night, dark and I can't see a thing! This causes me to have the giggles, which wakes Trevor up. In a round about way the test does work as I now know that he is awake! He does not seem to have a sense of humour at this time of the morning and suggests that I go to the front room and leave him to sleep!

Unfortunately my steroid sense of humour comes with me and I reflect on having a picket line. My union is to be named Choriocarcinoma Recipients Appreciation Party (to be known as C.R.A.P.). I will need a campaign if there is to be an official picket line. I will call it patients emotional needs include steroids (P.E.N.I.S). This campaign is directed at a specialised nurse who refuses to give the extra steroids for medicinal purposes. I have decided to take the offer of the kennel from Trevor up and make it my campaign head quarters, and I am planning a petition which I will take to the department of health. So after I have finished this book a career in politics beckons! Think what I could save on the defence budget as with me you get 2 for the price of 1. By this I mean that you get a politician and Britain's nuclear deterrent rolled into one, what a vote winner!

After an unexciting journey to Charing Cross I am stunned to find my bed ready for me. This chemo is called PAC- PLAT, and it is not long before my chemo is started, the Piriton injected and I'm asleep. I wake to find Trevor gone to his accommodation and its late evening. Then I wake to find out that my chemo is finished and its 4:30am!

I have found out that my Beta HCG had made it to over 1000. No one told me and I had not asked. This is probably just as well, but I'm glad that I know now my level is dropping.

14*th* *February* 2007

Happy Valentines Day. There is the usual wait for the tablets which takes until lunchtime. As I'm not feeling too bad due to the extra steroids they have given me, we decide to visit the hospital restaurant before leaving. I must say that the food in the restaurant is very good; it's a shame they can't feed the sick people with the same quality of cuisine!

I leave the restaurant and wait for Trevor outside in the corridor. He leaves by another door and waits for me by the main entrance of the hospital. Sadly we both wait for each other. Then try and phone each other at the same time to find out where each of us is. Eventually we meet again. I'm on steroids, what's his excuse!

I get out of the door then return for a wee. I leave again and trip up in front of Myooran who has escaped the hospital for a sandwich. He tells me that he was coming to find me to tell me he is leaving. It will be sad to lose such a good doctor. He always has a smile on his face and has also managed to survive my sense of humour. He is very sweet when he says that he will miss me and hopes that I am well again soon. I give him a hug in my steroid induced state and float off towards the car.

Within a short while I am putting the seat back in the car, positioning my pillow and I'm asleep. Trevor wakes me up outside our house and I go to pick up my handbag. At this point I realise that picking up my handbag from the hospital toilets would have been a better idea! There then follows numerous phone calls to cancel all my bank cards, which have not been used yet. Trevor contacts the security office at Charing Cross to see if my handbag has been handed in, but no luck. The thing that gets me to most is not that I left my handbag behind or the cancelling of all the cards, it's the fact that I can't go and buy another bag. I am now banned from places where there are large groups of people who could have infections. Internet shopping just does not do it for me. So I have to resort to giving orders to my children as to what I need, one bag, one purse and a diary (my needs are few!).

I have to get some replacement drugs from the doctor, but my medical exemption card was in my bag, so I now need to sort that as well. I don't think I will forget my handbag again for a while!

Beta HCG 26

19th February 2007

I have spent the last few days in bed, which seems to be how this chemo regime is going to be. I have gone from feeling limp to floppy. The pain of my joints swelling at times is almost unmanageable. After the last tramadol induced experience I am trying to take milder pain killers during the day and a tramadol at night. This however does not relieve all the pain during the day and with the sickness and fatigue all I do is just lie down. I am aware that my sides are getting sore, so I try to sit up for a while as I don't want to get bed sores as well. It would be very useful to discuss with my doctor my pain relief but when you just want to lie down this is not possible. I'll put it on my 'to do' list!

Today I am determined to go out for a while. Trevor and I have a cunning plan. We drive to Dawlish and get a pasty. Then drive to the top of the cliffs above Teignmouth and sit in the car and eat. The rain is falling onto the windscreen and its blowing a gale, but I don't care. This is one of those times when I realise how special life is.

Of course there is the blood test and I have to get some medication for the thrush in my mouth, but as Trevor says "it's all part of it"!

I do need to mention here that I feel the need to e-mail Linda having read the information she has given me about the latest chemo regime I am on. I have just read that the chemo will affect my ability to father a child. Well I'm shocked, as for Trevor, he is in a foetal position in a corner of the room, sobbing. He is grieving the loss of being able to experience the joys of giving birth. I wonder if we will be offered

IVF or will we be caught in the NHS postcode lottery. If so, where can I buy a ticket? I will await her reply.

20ᵗʰ *February 2007*

Linda has rang. She is pleading innocence over the fathering a child information and thinks I could be mad! The good news is that she has managed to arrange for the PAC-E chemo to be given in Exeter, with the first one being next Tuesday. The only difference is in Exeter they do this chemo as an overnight stay, not a day case. I don't mind as one less journey to London a month is great.

I have spent the afternoon at the Force cancer centre in a looking good, feeling better make up session. Those people who will admit to calling me a friend know that I don't wear make up, however I don't normally have cancer so I thought I've have a go.

There were about 12 woman all having some kind of cancer treatment in one room with a couple of make up consultants and 2 assistants. The room seemed a little tense until one of the make up consultants asked if anyone needed a hair clip to hold their hair back from their face. This is when I realised that I was the only one wearing a hat. So I took my hat off to reveal my bald head and said "I don't think I'll bother!" This seemed to break the ice and from then on it was a great afternoon. I did find some of the make up difficult to use due to the lack of feeling in my fingers. At one point while trying to put on some eyeliner I began to look like someone from the rocky horror show. I do not have a problem with asking for help, so managed to look almost human after the session. I can't wait for the next one.

21*st* *February 2007*

I have decided to buy a DVD recorder as I don't seem to be able to stay awake after 9:00pm and there are programmes I want to watch.

This is not going to be simple as I can't go shopping and Trevor is technologically dysfunctional! So I am resorting to the internet. After searching numerous web sites I have found the one I would like. You just know there is a but, well here it comes. The shop only has this model in a store 20 miles from our home! So we decide to make a lunch of it. We are becoming the Darby and Joan of the cancer world and sit in the car eating lunch while looking out over a football field. At least it's not the four walls of home again. Of course we get the mad woman in the car next to us. There we were enjoying a quiet lunch when a small silver cars pulls up beside us. She winds her window down, which seems a strange thing to do when it's 8 degrees and then turns her radio up. We do not wish to share her taste in radio broadcasting. Her head appears to be at a jaunty angle to the point of Trevor asking me if she has died. We decide to leave quickly and make our escape before the excitement gets too much for us.

After purchasing the DVD recorder it's time to return home, as the fatigue is setting in again.

I have managed to misread my brother's text inviting us to coffee and cakes on our way home and I think he is coming to see me. So half an hour after the suggested meeting time he rings to find out where we are. Plan b, Caroline brings George, Harry and the cakes to me. Within half an hour of Caroline and the boys leaving I'm asleep. Then awake, bath and bed by 6 o'clock.

The DVD can wait for another day to be set up!

22ⁿᵈ *February 2007*

The morning blood test has been completed with extra pain. Because of the planned insertion of the picket line, I am not allowed to have blood taken from the middle of my arm. All blood samples are being taken from the back of my hand, which really hurts. I also now have green and yellow bruises on the back of my hand. Becky and Vicky are sure that it is only a matter of time before I am picked up by the police as a drug addict!

This theory is compounded by the arrival of Colleen who has brought me some mushrooms which look like magic mushrooms. Is she in partnership with my children? Is there a conspiracy against me? Am I paranoid? (Don't answer that!).

I have decided to cook a meal tonight for Sally. This involves military planning to ensure that I have enough energy to make it to the end of the evening.

Manoeuvre plans are as follows;

Trevor dispatched to buy the ingredients, as I can't go to supermarkets.
Pudding is to be made in the afternoon, so I can have a rest before the meal
Main course to be prepared in afternoon, so I can have more rest
Main course to be cooked in 30 minutes, so I can have lots more rest

Well the rest worked and I even managed to stay awake during the meal. I now need more rest before planning another meal!

The DVD can wait until another day to be set up.

Beta HCG now 7

23rd *February 2007*

I have arranged a massage today. I still feel very tired, but a massage is worth making the effort for. Having said that I can report that today was the first time that a massage hurt. I think that my body is taking such a pounding from all the chemo that it is sore all over.

I return home for lunch and very soon I am asleep on the sofa. I am sound asleep when Trevor wakes me up. I could have done with another hour's sleep, but we have arranged to meet a retired publisher this afternoon, and I don't want to miss it having already missed one time by being taken into hospital. So I'm up, blurry eyed and doing a good impression of the ministry of silly walks.

The meeting was a real joy. Len, a retired publishers' agent is charming and funny and reminds me of Spike Milligan. His friend Jill, who introduced us to each other, became Lens double act and we laughed our way through 2 hours.

Len says that I need to get an agent, I'm now going to be wearing a red rose and carrying a copy of the Times, so MI5 will recognise me. Seriously I am now on the hunt to find an agent to get this book published and if you are reading this now, then I have been successful, if youre not reading this then!!!!

It's early bed tonight and had we have set up the DVD I would be recording he programmes that I will be sleeping through later.

The DVD will be set up another day

24th *February 2007*

A day spent mainly in bed I think. Well I know it will be by the lack of energy, and my inability to move.

The morning is a chance for me to think about how to set up the DVD. However it appears that it is not only my body that does not move, but also my brain. I can normally set up electrical equipment without having to think too hard. Now I don't seem to be able to think through any problems or be able to sequence events.

This does frustrate me, as I am normally good at sorting out problems. So I give up and get Trevor to phone an engineer to help. This frustrates me even more as now I am going to have to pay someone to do something that I would normally do.

By the afternoon I have worked out how to set the DVD up. However don't get too excited on my behalf as I will be getting Trevor to set it up in the bedroom as there are too many wires behind the front room TV for me to think about. So although we will have a DVD it will be in the wrong room!

The evening arrives and so do Vicky, Richard and the dog. I had earlier invited them to tea. It seemed a good idea at the time, and it is lovely to see them, but I forgot how tired I am. I am finding the more fatigued I get, the less noise I can manage. This is one of these times. So after tea, I retire to bed, and snuggle into the duvet.

The DVD is working!

26th *February 2007*

Up with the lark to make some cakes. I'm not sure why I had to get up early to make cakes, it just happened.

Lesson one of the day is that when you can't feel the end of your fingers, you do not remove hot cakes from the baking tin! Luckily I realised what I was doing after removing the second cake and stopped before burning the ends of my fingers.

The first appointment of the day is with Melissa, who seems happier to see the cakes than me. I am a disappointment to Melissa as I only have 15 out of 16 side effect mentioned in the information Linda has given me on my chemo regime. Melissa says I am a failure for not getting 100%. Well who needs diarrhoea anyway!

Second appointment is with Jacky, the incontinence nurse. I tell her that I am a relapsed cancer addict. We agree that there is still hope for me, but with everything going on in my life at present I should manage the incontinence as it is for the time being. There will be time after the chemo to sort my problem out.

I tell Jacky how difficult it has been for the past 3 days. You see I have had to measure my fluid input and output. The input part was no problem. As for the output, well have you ever tried to wee into a jug that you can't feel with your finger while balancing on feet that you can't feel either! Talk about a circus act!

Third appointment of the day is with Kieran to talk about my pain relief when my joints swell after chemo. Mild pain killers are not enough. Tramadol is an experience best not repeated. So it's oral morphine for me now. I can't wait for this one!

I also need to report that although the DVD is working, I failed to programme it to record properly. I now have a quarter of a play on disc.

The report card of the day reads Nikki Coombs could do better!

27ʰ February 2007

Well what a day! Have the nursing profession got it in for me? I have been good! but they tried to give me the wrong Chemo treatment!

There I was sat in the dayroom of the ward, when in comes the nurse and says ' we'll start your chemo here as your bed is not ready and you have nine hours of treatment' 'no this is only a six hour treatment' I reply. 'I had the nine hour PAC-PLAT treatment last time, this time it is the PAC-E treatment. She checks her records, checks my chemo book and leaves to sort it out.

Within 10 mins I have my Exeter consultant sat beside me apologising and showing me the letters from Linda in London. I can see how it had happened and as you would have guessed by now take it all in my stride as this is how my life happens around me. I do think that if everything went to plan, I would not be able to cope and would have to be sectioned under the mental health act!

I get my right chemo, which has the usual effect of me being wide awake one minute and fast asleep the next. I get a bed in the ward and realise that my chemo will not finish until 9:45pm and I am still in my day clothes. As I am not Houdini I will have to wait until after the chemo has finished to put my pyjamas on as there is no way I can get my top off while I have a drip in my arm.

I settle down to await the finish off my chemo when the nurse comes and asks me how I feel. 'Not too bad' I reply. It turns out they have an emergency coming in and need a bed. As I was an emergency only a few weeks back, I am happy to give up my hospital bed and replace it with my own bed. So I ring Trevor and ask him to come and get me at 10:00pm.

Can my life get anymore exciting?

Next week 2007

And as if by magic a week has gone by!

I do have to say that I am not having the time of my life! I have spent the last week mostly in bed on morphine. The time it takes to recover after each chemo is getting longer and harder to manage.

Although the morphine takes away the pain I can still feel my joints are sore and my muscles are tender. I am no longer floating round the ceiling as I was on the tramadol, but my speech seems to be impaired and I keep using all the right letters just in the wrong order, so if anyone has a bas garbaque for sale let me know. I have also described myself as feeling fimp and loopy, which is a new medical term!

Oh joy I have woken up in the middle of the night and I have spots. They are up the inside of my arms, across my back and a few over my chest, just for good measure. I phone to get advice. I have to take some piriton and come into the hospital in Exeter and see a doctor tomorrow. Well I haven't been to hospital for 6 days and I would not want withdrawal symptoms would I?

So off to hospital I go to see a doctor. I have blood taken and await the results. Within an hour I am called back to the doctor. My blood results are fine, but I am allergic to the chemo. Well that's a new one for me! Mind you with all the side effects I have had its not surprising. This does not mean that they will stop giving me the chemo it just means more piriton.

Just completing a small task takes so much effort that I have to stop and sit down at regular intervals, and walking up my garden steps requires oxygen. I am also getting frustrated at not being able to do much my body may have slowed, but my mind still has things to do.

The good news is that my HCG level is back to 3 and I will find out on Tuesday when I have chemo in Charing Cross how many more chemo's I have to go.

10th March 2007

I am determined to go out today. I have to get to Plymouth by next Saturday to pick up Becky's birthday present, so that's where we are going. I know when I get onto the car that it will be to much for me, but I am not telling Trevor that as he won't take me else. I manage the journey of 45 minutes to Plymouth, A very short walk around the pannier market. Then we pick up Becky's tickets, and I'm exhausted to the point of collapse. The planned pasty on the sea front is abandoned in favour of home and bed. Half way home I need to eat, so Trevor finds somewhere to pull of the road. We stop just long enough to eat, then we are on our way again.

I fall into bed and cry. It was far too much for me. I am worried how I will manage the trip to London in 3 days time. I ache so much that I take morphine. I am scared that the chemo will be finishing soon and I will be back in limbo land again, waiting to see if the HCG level rises again. There is nothing right, and nothing that Trevor says will make it alright. So I cry more. Then I fall asleep.

I wake an hour later and just lie still, feeling sorry for myself. Well I am ill you know!

Lots of next weeks
Yes it's been a while since I've written anything, but I do have a good excuse. You see although I have little feeling in my fingers and toes, I do have pain in them. Therefore pressing the keys on the keyboard hurts. That's my excuse and I'm sticking to it.

So it's time to update you on what's been happening.

Yes I did make it to London and also for my final Chemo in Exeter.

I have had one of those conversations where there is something that I can't say, well just let me tell you about it. I go to clinic in Charing Cross hospital where the subject of my post chemo check date is discussed. Linda wants to set the date for the 7th of May. I don't want to go on this date because I have arranged a special birthday present for Trevor to say thank you for all he has done for me. This will involve him joining my brother, Simon and Jen's husband, Rob in a white knuckle ride in a Ferrari, around a race track, with a racing driver. It is not Trevor's birthday yet so I can't tell them as Trevor is sat beside me! So I tell Linda that Jen's son might get to the final of the FA vase and would then be playing at the new Wembley stadium on the 13th of May. So the date is made for the 14th of May, and Linda is looking at me with a puzzled look on her face. I return home the next day and email Linda to tell her why I was avoiding the 7th of May, and then text Jen and ask to tell her son that there is no pressure but he'd better get to Wembley!

Each time I have another Chemo the side effects are getting worse. I am now unable to get up for 7 days after each Chemo session and can't wait till this is all over. I am taking morphine for the pain of the side effects, then laxatives for the effects of the side effects, side effects medicine!

I am also getting anxious, as it is coming up to the time when the chemo has stopped and limbo land till the six week post chemo check happens. I have been here before and as you know it was not a success before.

I am so exhausted that accomplishing just one small task in a day is an achievement.

However, the humour has not left me!

Trevor has been teak oiling the outdoor table and chairs. He is offering to oil my legs to give me a tan as I am not allowed out in the sun in case I burn.

Linda has put me on some new tablets to help with the pain in my fingers and toes. I have now read the side effects of the tablets and I am concerned in case my testicles swell and I have hair loss! The question is how will I know if I have hair loss or will it have a reverse effect and make my hair grow?

Becky has returned from a holiday in Las Vegas. You would think that as her mother has been unwell a great present would be in order. I get a red tee shirt with 'I need supervision' written on it. No you don't have to agree with her! I am thinking of going into business selling this tee shirt as I have has so many offers for it I could have sold loads.

I have decided to have a party to celebrate my birthday, so I send out invitations to some of my family and friends to invite them to my 'I've made it to my birthday party'. Colleen rings me and tells me that she is not keen on the title of my party, because if she knows that is was going to be such a close battle with the cancer she would have chosen what she wanted from my house before. I still let her come to the party!

My mobility seems to be getting worse even though my chemo has now finished. My hips and knees are ceasing up and I am waking up at night in pain. After taking this over with doctor Kieran I am back on pain killers and to top it all my face has exploded into a rash. So I am also back on antibiotics.

Colleen has kindly lent us her house while she is away. So I am able to look at a different four walls for a change, however this does not last long as she has failed to install a stair lift, and due to my mobility being limited at present going up and down her windy staircase is the equivalent of climbing Mount Everest! So we depart for home early. So if you get cancer, live in a bungalow!

My mood seems to being dropping the closer I get to my post chemo check up. I know that my HCG levels have remained normal, but until I hear Professor Seckl tell me I'm cancer free, I can't rest. While discussing with Trevor how I feel he tells me that until the final scans results come back the professor won't be able to write me off! He has such a way with words, although I do understand what he is saying.

Sunday 13th May 2007

It's the day before the post chemo check up. Yes Jen's son has made it to the Wembley final, so we are meeting her and a minibus full of her family and friends at Exeter service station to travel up. This also means that we have finally completed our service station challenge. We have visited every service station between here and Charing Cross on the M5 and M4. Marks out of ten will now be allocated to all service stations, but for fear of being sued if I tell you the results, I will have to kill you!

We are followed by the minibus to Wembley, as we have Jane Satnav. She becomes quite stroppy as the staff at Wembley have closed off the entrance that she wants us to drive in and keep telling us to turn around when possible. We pull up and ask a steward which way we need to go to get into the disabled parking, 'around the back' he replies. Well when you don't know if you are at the back or the front of somewhere this is not useful! We eventually find the back, which seemed like the side, then drove around the front! Yes we were confused too!

The football match was great as they won 3-1. This was after a nail biting finish which caused me to tell Jen that if after all the chemo I have had, I now died of a heart attack it would be her fault!

We spend the night at the visitor's accommodation eating kebabs and watching television. I'm exhausted so it's early bed for me and no problem with sleeping.

Monday 14th May 2007

Breakfast in the hospital canteen and then off to clinic.

I walk into the consulting room to be greeted by Linda making a strange face. Apparently it's nothing to do with me! The student doctor had just given her a sour sweet. I will fill in her application to the gurning competition later.

My HCG is still normal; however it would not be that simple would it? After being hit with a hammer and tickled with a tissue and rubber glove (they couldn't find the tissues at first!) I still have problems with the feeling in my fingers and toes, plus I have sluggish reflexes down my left hand side. So I'm not to be written off yet. I am to return in 6 weeks and be referred to another specialist for my fingers and toes.

Linda takes 6 tubes of blood from me and tells me she is optimistic this time. Well I'll go for that. She has arranged for my last scan to be brought forward, which is great. So it's off for a CT scan next.

The CT scan gives me the opportunity to wear one of the wonderful hospital gowns. My name is called and I go off for the scan with a nurse.

Trevor is sat in the waiting room when a man and woman arrive. The woman in a loud voice says to the man 'do you know, some people like coming to hospital, they must be sick'

CT scan over and it's time for the MRI scan, it must be my lucky day! 25 mins inside a tube and I'm done. You guessed it I can't go until I have a blood test result which takes another hour.

We finally escape and we are on our way home. I'm fairly happy with what has happened today, but I am sad that I haven't been written off.

Speaking of written off, I feel it's a good time to finish writing now as my cancer levels have remained normal for a while and I am only dealing with lingering side effects.

So how to sign off?

Well I'm off to live for the rest of my life. It won't be the same life as before as the cancer has changed the way I look at life, but live it to the full I will.

I'm not going to get all philosophical now. The only way I can think of to finish this is where I began, so here goes.

So thanks Kieran and goodnight.

p.s thought you might like an update. My HCG is still normal and it is now 12 weeks since I had chemo, and I have just been told that I am cured. Even I'm optimistic now!

I have seen another Professor about the numbness in my fingers and toes and my joint pains. After various tests, which included sticking needles in my feet (which will hurt you thinking about that more than it did me actually having it done!). He has concluded that I was moderately abnormal! Trevor is disputing the moderate part, my brother wants to know how much the professor is paid as he could have told me that for less, and Linda is hysterical.

What the professor means is that for my condition of peripheral neuropathy I am in the moderate range and having the condition is not normal. Well at least I understand him!

The aches and pains should go, but in months not weeks and only time will tell whether the feeling will return in my fingers and toes, but hey, I'm alive

The best news of all, as far as I am concerned is that I have dandruff and I am proud of it! This means that I also have hair, which is about 1" long and curly. Jane has offered me some head lice, but this is too much excitement to bear, so I have declined her offer!

So this time it really is
thanks Kieran and goodnight.

GLOSSARY OF TERMS

Medical terminology	Our terminology
Beta HCG	HSBC
FBC (full blood count)	KFC
GCSF injections	GCSE
Hysterectomy with ovaries removed.	Full English
Hysterectomy without ovaries removed.	Continental
Domperidone (anti-sickness tablets)	Dom perignon
Diclofenac (pain killer)	Diplomatic
Intrathecal room	In the cathedral room
Civas (where the chemo is made up)	Sea bass
Ganesitron (anti-sickness tablets)	Gravel stone
Gabapentin (fingers and toes tablets)	Gabby Roslyn
Pyridoxine (vitamin B6)	Peroxide
Nortriptyline (fingers and toes tablets)	Norah Batty

About the Author

Nikki Coombs has lived and worked in Devon all her life. She is married to Trevor and has two adult daughters.

She had worked for most of her life in the caring professions and never dreamt that she would one day be needing people to care for her.

At the age of 45 she was diagnosed with a rare form of cancer called, Choriocarcinoma.

At that point her life turned upside down. She learnt how to get through one day at a time and face each challenge as it was thrown at her.

Although she has always had an 'alternative' sense of humour, she never thought she would be relying on it to see her through the toughest times of her life.

Nikki never aspired to write a book, in fact she vowed never to write anything more than a letter to her doctor. But 49,000 words later, here's her book!

Printed in the United Kingdom
by Lightning Source UK Ltd.
124907UK00001B/46-90/A